W9-CSD-835

WITHDRAWN

Improving
Your Memory

DATE DUE

Improving Your Memory

How to Remember What You're Starting to Forget

4TH EDITION

Janet Fogler and
Lynn Stern

Johns Hopkins University Press
Baltimore

9 8 7 6 5 4 3 2 1

Johns Hopkins University Press
2715 North Charles Street
Baltimore, Maryland 21218-4363
www.press.jhu.edu

Library of Congress Cataloging-in-Publication Data

Fogler, Janet.
  Improving your memory : how to remember what you're starting to forget /
Janet Fogler and Lynn Stern. — Fourth edition.
      pages cm
  ISBN 978-1-4214-1570-3 (pbk. : alk. paper) — ISBN 1-4214-1570-4
(pbk. : alk. paper) — ISBN 978-1-4214-1571-0 (electronic) — ISBN 1-4214-1571-2
(electronic)   1. Memory—Age factors.   2. Memory in old age.
3. Mnemonics.   I. Stern, Lynn, 1949–   II. Title.
  BF724.85.M45F64 2014
  153.1'22–dc23   2014008681

A catalog record for this book is available from the British Library.

*Special discounts are available for bulk purchases of this book. For more
information, please contact Special Sales at 410-516-6936 or
specialsales@press.jhu.edu.*

Johns Hopkins University Press uses environmentally friendly book
materials, including recycled text paper that is composed of at least
30 percent post-consumer waste, whenever possible.

Contents

IV Techniques for Improving Your Memory

Acknowledgments

We would like to express our appreciation and gratitude to all of our colleagues at the University of Michigan Medical Center's Turner Geriatric Clinic. We especially thank Ruth Campbell for her early recognition of the importance of addressing age-related memory concerns and for her encouragement and support through the years. Mary Rumman has worked with us to offer memory improvement classes in the community. Tami Remington provided us with the latest information on medications that may have an impact on memory. Jennifer Howard, Barbara Betts Swartz, and Maire Ready updated the appendix on Alzheimer's disease. We appreciate all of them for their contributions.

The W. K. Kellogg Foundation sponsored our first research in this area as well as the memory improvement programs we offered throughout the country.

Our editor, Jackie Wehmueller, and copy editor, Michele Callaghan, have given us generously of their time and talents. Their thoughtful comments have helped make this edition even better.

Scott and Neal have brainstormed memory solutions, eaten postponed meals, and as always, given us their support.

Last, we owe a tremendous debt of gratitude to the hundreds of people who have been members of our memory improvement classes. You have provided us with questions, solutions, and humorous examples. Thanks for the inspiration and fun!

Part I

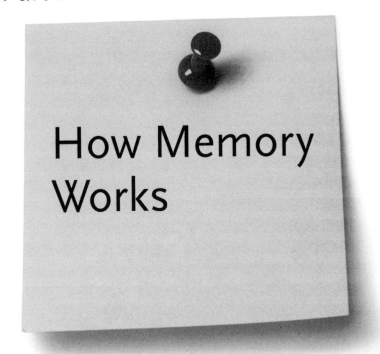

How Memory Works

1

You Can Improve Your Memory

> Our heads may be small, but they are as full
> of memories as the sky may sometimes be full of
> swarming bees, thousands and thousands of
> memories, of smells, of places, of little things that
> happened to us and which came back, unexpectedly,
> to remind us who we are.
>
> —*Alexander McCall Smith*

Since 2005, when we wrote the previous edition of this book, technology has exploded with "fixes" for common memory lapses. There is a reason for this. People of all ages want to avoid the consequences of forgetting. Car lights, space heaters, and coffee pots can turn themselves off. Thermostats can be programmed to adjust the heat and air conditioning automatically. Smartphones and devices help us keep track of appointments, phone numbers, and e-mail addresses and alert us with alarms when it's time to do something.

But, we are still anxious when words and names stay stuck on the tips of our tongues; we still misplace items and forget to do things; memory is still affected by illness, overwork, or mood. We are more than ever challenged by a bombardment of information and overextended schedules. More than ever we talk with each other and in the media about failing memories, and we wonder what to do about them.

The information about memory and the memory improvement techniques in *Improving Your Memory* will help you understand how memory works, why you forget, and how memory changes with age. By combining this understanding with the basic tips and techniques described in this book, you can improve your memory.

The basics still apply:

- No one can remember everything. We have to make choices about where to put our effort.
- The first step is to pay attention to the things we want to remember.
- There are techniques for remembering the things that are most important to each of us.
- We need to keep up with mental, physical, and social activities without overwhelming ourselves. If we establish good habits—such as keeping lists, returning items to their proper place, and reducing clutter in our homes— we can relieve the clutter in our minds.

EXAMPLES

Barbara works part-time in a toy store, is on the board of the library, and never misses her nephew's soccer games. Recently, she was embarrassed when she ran into an acquaintance and could not call her by name. A week later Barbara walked out of the shopping mall and couldn't remember where she had parked her car. The following month, she realized she was losing track of the cast of characters in a novel she was reading. Then she completely forgot a lunch date with a good friend. Barbara was extremely worried, especially when she thought of her uncle, who had been diagnosed with Alzheimer's disease.

Carl is an engineer at a water treatment plant. Last month he couldn't remember if he had changed the oil in his car or just thought about doing it. He missed the turn to the recreation center and didn't realize it until several streets passed by. He couldn't remember where in the garage he had hidden a house key. Carl wondered whether the problem was his memory or the stress he was under at work.

You and your friends may have had experiences similar to Carl's and Barbara's, and you, too, may have concerns about your memory. People of all ages complain about forgetting, but, as people grow older, they often worry when they cannot remember a familiar name or where they parked the car. Memory does change as people age, but almost everyone can improve memory with training and practice.

Here are some common complaints shared by friends and clients. (And we confess that we have made these statements, too!)

- I went into a room and couldn't remember why.
- I couldn't remember what I wanted to ask the doctor.
- I hid a birthday gift for my wife and couldn't remember where.
- I had to pay a late fee because I didn't pay the electric bill on time.
- I forgot to bring my camera on a trip.
- I went to the store for milk and got everything but.
- I forgot how to enter a new contact on my smartphone.

- I forgot my sister's birthday.
- I forgot whether I took my medication.
- I heard a great joke, but I can't remember what it was.

If you have had any of these experiences, you can benefit from this book. We will teach you how to recognize and address common memory problems by discussing how memory works; how memory changes with age; factors that affect memory; and concrete strategies for improving memory.

To make this book as useful as possible, we include many suggestions about what you can do in everyday life. Examples and pen-and-paper exercises demonstrate memory concepts and techniques.

You will find this book most helpful if you read it carefully, do all the exercises, and experiment with the strategies in your daily life. We can't promise that you will never have memory lapses again, but we know that you can make positive changes in your memory and have fun doing it.

2

Understanding the Components of Memory

It's a poor sort of memory that only works backwards.
—*Lewis Carroll*

"I just can't remember anymore!"

"My memory has gotten so bad!"

If you find yourself saying things like this, you may have given in to the myth that aging and memory loss go hand in hand. When people believe this myth, they may even stop *trying* to remember. But we know—and studies show—that memory can be improved with training and practice.

To improve the memory process, it helps to understand how memory works. Although the brain is not understood nearly as well as the heart or the circulatory system, memory experts have devised a way to visualize how we remember. They often describe the memory process as having three components.

1. **Sensory input,** the first component of the memory process, is the mind's brief recognition of what we see, hear, touch, smell, or taste. We are constantly surrounded by sights and sounds, and we immediately discard much of what we see and hear. There is no need for us to record it. When we pay attention to a sensory impression, however, the sight or sound, the

touch, smell, or taste enters the second component of memory, known as "working memory."

2. **Working memory** may be equated with conscious thought: the small amount of material that can be held in the mind at any given moment. Most experts believe that working memory can hold no more than six or seven items. This material will be discarded in five to ten seconds unless it is either continually repeated or stored in long-term memory.

An example of information that is held in working memory and generally discarded without being stored is a telephone number. Say you look up a phone number, make the call, and can't reach the person. Once you hang up, you may realize that you have already forgotten the number you just called. This is a good demonstration of how information disappears from working memory after only a brief time.

In another example, say you hear a nutritionist state that there are eleven grams of fat in one tablespoon of butter. You are surprised at how high this number is. Later, however, you can't recall or even recognize that number in a multiple choice question on a television quiz show.

As you read this book, keep in mind this important fact—not all information that registers in working memory gets stored in long-term memory.

3. **Long-term memory,** the memory bank, is the largest component of the memory system. Its storage space is practically limitless. A common misconception is that long-term memory refers to events that occurred a long time ago. In fact, however, long-term memory holds information that was learned as recently as a few minutes ago and as long ago as many decades. This storage space may hold items as varied as

- Your name
- What happened an hour ago

- Where you spent last Thanksgiving
- The information needed to drive a car
- The smell of baking cookies
- An image of your high school math teacher
- The multiplication tables
- A song from the 1980s

Thus, long-term memory refers to any information that is no longer in conscious thought but is stored for possible recollection.

Here are two examples of how the memory process works in daily life.

EXAMPLES

You are doing your weekly shopping at the local grocery store. There are many items on the shelves that make sensory impressions on you. You see the colors of the packages, smell the bakery products, and hear the many sounds around you. These sensory impressions, however, may or may not register in conscious thought.

You pause in the produce department and consider what fruit to serve in a salad. You glance at a papaya, a fruit you have never tried, and notice that it is very expensive. If you then move on, you will probably not recall the papaya in any detail. The impression of the papaya has entered working memory (conscious thought) but has not necessarily been stored in long-term memory.

If you pay more attention to the papaya, however, by noting its shape, color, and texture, smelling its fragrance, feeling its ripeness, and even thinking about what it might taste like or how you could prepare it, the image and knowledge of that fruit will probably be transferred into long-term memory. This

A MODEL FOR HOW MEMORY WORKS
The flow of information through the three components of memory

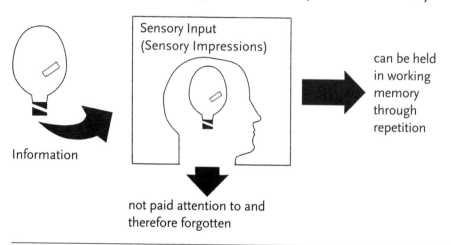

Sensory Input
(Sensory Impressions)

can be held
in working
memory
through
repetition

Information

not paid attention to and
therefore forgotten

information will be available for retrieval in the future, for example, when you see a recipe that includes papaya as an ingredient.

You are addressing envelopes announcing a shower for your niece. You have a list of names but no home addresses. Your task is to look up the addresses and transfer the names and addresses to the envelopes. As you handle the phone book, your senses take in the feel of the book, the pattern of the names on a given page, and the sound of pages turning (or the feel of the pages in your hand). These sensory impressions may or may not register in working memory.

You find Laura Adam's name and copy her address to an envelope: 4276 Woodlawn St., Chelsea, Michigan. This information has entered working memory. You hold it in your mind for the few seconds needed to address the envelope. If you are not familiar with this street, you are unlikely to store this infor-

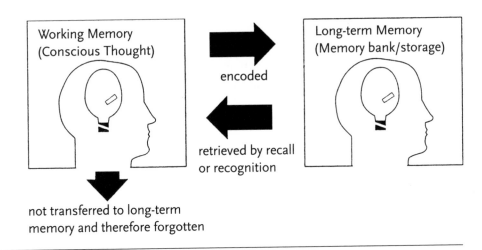

Working Memory (Conscious Thought)

encoded

Long-term Memory (Memory bank/storage)

retrieved by recall or recognition

not transferred to long-term memory and therefore forgotten

mation in long-term memory. After a few moments, you probably won't even remember the name of the street.

If you note that Woodlawn Street is in your son's neighborhood, however, and wonder whether your son knows Laura, you are more likely to transfer the information to long-term memory and think of her as you drive down Woodlawn on the way to your son's house.

Even though we have presented the components of memory as if new information always flows from sensory memory to working memory to long-term memory, it is possible for information that has not registered in conscious thought to be stored in long-term memory. In certain situations you may remember things without realizing that they have entered your awareness. For example, you may not be consciously aware of all of the people sitting in the doctor's waiting room with you, but when a man comes in and asks if you have seen a woman in a wheelchair, you recall that the nurse took a woman in a wheelchair into an exam room.

Now that you have learned about the components of memory, you have a framework for recognizing why you may remember or forget certain things. Throughout the book, additional information—such as factors that affect memory and techniques to improve memory—will be related to this chapter's description of the components of the memory process.

3

How We Remember

To observe attentively is to remember distinctly.
—*Edgar Allan Poe*

Although we may be frustrated when we forget, the truly remarkable aspect of memory is the vast amount of information we are able to store and recall. When a classmate at a reunion asks a question like "Do you remember the day John Arbec got lost at the science museum?" most of us are, in fact, able to remember that incident!

Remembering depends on learning and storing information so that it can be retrieved at some future time. Thus, successful remembering requires two things:

1. Getting information solidly into long-term memory (we call this "encoding") and
2. Bringing needed information from long-term memory into working memory (we call this "retrieval").

Let's discuss what is involved in these two aspects of memory.

Encoding

The term "encoding" describes the process of getting information into long-term memory. Encoding consists of mental tasks, such as the following:

- Paying attention to something,
- Associating it with something already known,
- Analyzing the information for meaning, and
- Elaborating on the details.

Often these tasks are performed automatically, without any conscious effort on our part. These tasks give deeper meaning to the information and strengthen our chances of remembering it. Perhaps the easiest way to understand encoding is to look at how it works in everyday life.

EXAMPLE

Grant and Amy took a trip to Northern Michigan in 2010. During the weeklong vacation, they visited several beaches along the shore of Lake Michigan. On the most beautiful afternoon, they took a long walk along a deserted stretch of beach near Harbor Bay. They noticed that the rocky shoreline included multicolored pebbles and stones of all sizes worn perfectly smooth by the movement of the waves. They were amazed by the variety and number. This area was definitely different from the other beaches they had explored. They wondered what natural phenomenon had gifted this area with such beautiful stones. They collected some small stones to take home as souvenirs. They felt especially close to each other and to nature and went to their hotel feeling tired and content. Whenever they talk about this trip, they recall this day on the beach with great clarity. These memories are particularly strong, because they were encoded well and had both intellectual and emotional meaning.

Two tasks of encoding—attention and association—deserve some additional emphasis.

Attention

Remember when your mother used to tell you to "pay attention." She was right! Paying attention—the first step in the process of encoding information into long-term memory—is one of the tasks of working memory. At any moment, many pieces of information are competing for the attention of your working memory. You may need to make a conscious effort to focus your attention on what you want to remember. Keep in mind that the amount of material you can hold in your working memory is limited. You need to zero in on what is important. The following examples may remind you of a time when your attention wasn't focused properly.

EXAMPLES

A friend tells you to meet her for lunch at 12:00, and you make a note of the date, time, and place. You mistakenly arrive at the restaurant at 12:30 because you didn't pay attention when the time was discussed, and you wrote it down incorrectly. Next time, resolve to focus your attention on the details of time and place, repeat them out loud, and be sure you write them down correctly.

You were given directions to a new dentist's office, followed them carefully, and had no trouble finding it the first time. At the next visit, you assume that you will remember where to go. As you approach the area, you are confused about which high-rise building the office is in. You realize that you didn't pay enough attention to the location and the appearance of the building the first time. In the future, note some landmarks and descriptive features that will help you tell the buildings apart.

In both of these examples, you believed that you were paying enough attention to encode the information sufficiently, but clearly you weren't. Everyone has had this experience many times. We give superficial attention to a piece of information and then are frustrated when we can't remember it exactly. One of the simplest ways to improve your memory is to realize the importance of focusing your attention on what you really want to remember.

Since there are often many pieces of information competing for your attention, you may find that you have paid attention to the wrong thing and have missed what you really wanted to remember. For example, you're attending classes on memory improvement. All of a sudden, you realize that you've been staring at a woman's unusual clothing instead of paying attention to the teacher. The next day you can still recall the intricate beading on the woman's jacket but have no idea what to do for homework. In the future, when you forget something you wanted to remember, ask yourself if the problem was inadequate attention.

Association

Another aspect of encoding that deserves some explanation is association. Whether we are aware of it or not, new information is encoded by connecting it with other well-known and relevant information that already resides in long-term memory. This process is called "association." The easiest way to understand the concept of association is to look at how it happens effortlessly in daily life.

EXAMPLES

If you meet a new person, your memory of him may be encoded by making different associations. A friend introduced you at the theater, and you noticed his beautiful curly hair. He told you that he lives in Brooklyn and is a nurse. Thus, you could have made an association with these different classifications: curly-haired people, the theater where you met, other people who live in Brooklyn, the nursing profession, the woman who introduced him to you. In the future, thinking of any of these categories could trigger a recollection of your new acquaintance. When you see another curly-haired person or a nurse or go to the theater where you met, the experience may serve as a cue and you may think of the curly-haired nurse from Brooklyn. Although you made no effort to remember this person, your mind has made these associations on your behalf. Thanks, mind!

Suppose your granddaughter has recently been chosen to be on the high school field hockey team. You don't know anything about how the game is played or the equipment that's used, but you do know a lot about football. When your granddaughter explains the game and equipment to you, you automatically associate the new information about field size, scoring, timekeeping, and protective equipment with what you already know about football. Without any such associations, information about field hockey would be more difficult to encode. The next time you watch football on TV, you may think of your conversation with your granddaughter and remember that she has a field hockey game coming up.

Much association of new information is done unconsciously, but you can make a conscious effort to associate something you want to remember with something you already know. The more effort you put into creating these associations and the greater the number of cross-references available, the more likely you are to recall at will. Here are two examples of people who have made a conscious effort to associate something they want to remember with something they know well.

EXAMPLES

Amir's granddaughter is fascinated by the children's TV show *Sesame Street*. He recently bought a book about many of the Sesame Street characters. When she points to each character, wanting to know the name, Amir wants to be able to answer. He finds it difficult to differentiate between Bert and Ernie, two characters who are always seen together. In looking for ways to associate the names with the characters, he notices that Bert has a much bigger head. He thinks, "Bert—big! Both words begin with B. That's how I'll remember."

Anna has allergies to dust, animals, weeds, and grasses. At her doctor's office, she was given samples of two allergy medications to try. One of the medications was to be taken in the morning because it can disturb sleep; the other was to be taken at bedtime because it can cause sleepiness. When she got home, Anna had forgotten the doctor's instructions. Because there were no directions on the sample packages, Anna had to call the doctor's office for clarification. She decided to make a conscious effort to remember which medication was which. She noted that the daytime medicine was blue, and she associated the color with the blue daytime sky.

(If the daytime medicine was green, she could note that a green light means Go and think, "I get up and go in the morning, but not at night.")

Retrieval

Retrieval is the process of getting information from long-term memory into the conscious state of working memory. Most memory complaints center on the inability to bring information to mind on demand. In actuality, however, our ability to find a piece of information in our vast storehouse of memories and bring it to awareness is truly amazing and happens easily much of the time.

There are two ways you can retrieve information from long-term memory: recognition and recall.

Recognition is the perception of information that is presented to you as something or someone you already know. For example, you recognize the name of your friend's son when you hear it, but you could not come up with it on your own.

Recall is a self-initiated search of long-term memory for information you want. In most cases, recall is more challenging than recognition. Recall of information is difficult, because you must find one piece of information among the millions that are stored in long-term memory.

For example, say you want to talk about your former neighbor and you search your memory bank to recall the name. Although you know you would recognize the name, recalling it far more difficult.

When you say, "I can't remember," you usually mean, "I can't recall." It may be hard to recall the name of a TV show, but you may recognize the name of the show easily when you see it in the programming schedule.

When a friend of ours had trouble recalling the name of a new medication, she laughingly said, "I wish this were a multiple choice question."

✱ EXERCISE: RECALL

To answer the following questions, you are required to recall the information from long-term memory. If you find this task difficult, try to see if you can recognize the correct answers to the questions as they are asked again on page 28.

1. What is the capital city of Illinois?
2. Who played Dorothy in the movie *The Wizard of Oz?*
3. Who ran for president against Jimmy Carter in 1976?
4. Who was the mayor of New York City on 9/11/2001?

See page 149 for answers.   ✱

Sometimes recall of information is triggered by a cue. A **cue** is an event, thought, picture, word, sound, smell, or something else that triggers the retrieval of information from long-term memory. For example, you may be able to recall the last name of your neighbor when prompted with the first name. This triggering information, the first name, is a cue.

People often say, "I can't remember names, but I never forget a face." We remember faces easily because they present themselves for recognition. Remembering names, in contrast, involves recall of information from long-term memory, for which the face is only a cue. (Recently the media have called attention to a condition called "prosopagnosia," or face blindness, which impairs a person's ability to recognize faces, even the face of a spouse or another person very closely connected to the person with the condition. This problem is different from not being able to remember the name of people even when you recognize their faces.)

When you are searching for a name or another piece of information, try thinking of related facts that may serve as cues. They will often trigger the desired piece of information. For example, if you are having trouble recalling what class you took last summer, you might think about where it was held, who was in the class with you, and other subjects you have taken in the past.

4

Why We Forget

Remembrance of things past is not necessarily the remembrance of things as they were.

—*Marcel Proust*

No one can remember everything. An essential part of the memory process is making decisions about what information is valuable to you and worth the effort to encode it. Is it really critical to spend energy encoding the name of a woman who occasionally teaches your exercise class when she is only an infrequent substitute? It might be better to choose to learn the name of your neighbor's new baby.

Most people feel very frustrated and even embarrassed when they have to say, "I've forgotten." Rather than blame a faulty memory, consider instead that there are some good reasons for not remembering.

1. **Some information never gets into the memory bank.** It gets only as far as sensory input or working memory. Why? You didn't pay attention to it. You didn't really hear it. You didn't understand it. You didn't care enough to remember it. You got distracted by something else. You didn't need to remember it.

2. Memories that do enter the memory bank may be overlaid with subsequent similar information that makes the original memory irretrievable. People often describe their inadequacies in memory by saying, "I can't even remember what I ate for breakfast yesterday." If you eat similar types of breakfast food day after day, you may forget what you ate on any particular morning, while the memory of the one time you ate a croissant baked by your French daughter-in-law remains firm.

3. Information for which you have few associations and little background knowledge is harder to remember. For example, if you are just a beginner at the game of bridge, you will find it hard to remember any particular hand dealt during an evening of play, but a bridge expert can accurately recall most of the cards in a particularly meaningful hand.

4. Some information may be remembered only when the proper cues are available, and those cues are not part of everyday life. For example, you may think you've forgotten many of your eighth-grade classmates until you find an old photo or go to a class reunion.

5. Who we are influences how we remember. Many people assume that their own memories are a true picture of what really happened, and they are upset or confused by the conflicting recollections of others. Personal differences can affect encoding of information and can influence the way we remember; our background, knowledge, training, stance on life, age, gender, and prejudices all have an impact on the way we interpret events and commit them to memory. When two people remember things differently, they may argue over who is "forgetting." In reality, the difference in recollection may be due to the differing views and experiences of the people involved.

6. Some pieces of remembered information may be assembled incorrectly. Pieces of information may be recalled but misassembled. For example, you described to your daughter a time when Uncle John fell out of a tree. She didn't remember the event, and you remarked that Aunt Rose didn't recall it, either. Several months later, you were surprised to hear your daughter tell the same story and say, "I heard this from Aunt Rose."

7. **Some memories fade away.** They are not readily available for all time. For example, if you studied a foreign language in high school, you may recall or recognize some of the vocabulary words you learned. However, you probably have no recollection of and wouldn't even recognize many other words you once knew.

5
Let's Review

Let's review some of the terms used to describe the memory process.

Sensory input: information that enters the brain through the five senses

Working memory: equated with conscious thought, the very small amount of information you can pay attention to at a given moment

Long-term memory: the accumulation of information that is not present in conscious thought but is stored for potential recollection

Encoding: the act of learning and storing information

Retrieval: the act of bringing information from long-term memory to conscious thought

Association: the connection between new information and what you already know

Recognition: the perception of information that is presented to you as something or someone you already know

Recall: a self-initiated search of long-term memory for information

Cue: the event, thought, picture, word, sound, smell, or something else that triggers the retrieval of information from long-term memory

Here are those questions again. Are they easier this time?

✳ EXERCISE: RECOGNITION

To answer the following questions, you are required to recognize the correct answers.

1. What is the capital city of Illinois?
   Chicago
   Peoria
   Springfield
   Champaign
2. Who played Dorothy in the movie *The Wizard of Oz*?
   Doris Day
   Judy Holliday
   Judy Garland
   Mary Martin
3. Who ran for president against Jimmy Carter in 1976?
   Ronald Reagan
   Gerald Ford
   Michael Dukakis
   George H. W. Bush
4. Who was the mayor of New York City on 9/11/2001?
   Michael Bloomberg
   Mario Cuomo
   Rudolph Giuliani
   Richard Daley

See page 149 for answers.   ✳

✳ EXERCISE: UNDERSTANDING THE MEMORY PROCESS

Complete the blanks in this scenario to test your understanding of the memory process. Use the words listed below.

Cue
Sensory input
Association
Encoding
Long-term memory
Working memory
Retrieval

When you go to the library and see a lot of colorful books on the "new books" shelf, the component of memory you are using is

_____.

You read through the titles and think about whether they interest you. These conscious thoughts occur in the component of memory called

_____.

Then you find a book by a favorite author, John Grisham. You take down the book, notice how long it is, read the back cover, think to yourself that it sounds familiar, and decide that you have read this book before. This process is called

_____.

The information about the book leaves your conscious thought and goes into the component of memory called

_____,

where it may be available for

_____

at another time. When you get home, you notice another of Grisham's books on your nightstand. This favorite book serves as a

_____

to remind you of the book in the library. The connection between the library book and your book at home is called

_____.

See page 149 for answers.   ✳

✳ EXERCISE: HOW MEMORY WORKS

True/False. Circle the answer.

T   F   1. Long-term memory refers to something that happened long ago.

T   F   2. All information in conscious thought becomes part of your long-term memory.

T   F   3. Sensory impressions may not register in conscious thought.

T   F   4. Associations are made both consciously and unconsciously.

T   F   5. One piece of new information can be associated with many different facts in your long-term memory.

T   F   6. When you are presented with a name that you perceive as something you know, this form of retrieval is called recognition.

T   F   7. Once information is encoded in long-term memory, it doesn't change.

See page 150 for answers.   ✳

Part II

How Memory Changes as We Age

6

What Changes?
What Doesn't?

How cruelly sweet are the echoes that start, when
memory plays an old tune on the heart!

—Eliza Cook

There are many myths about the inevitability of memory loss
as people age. The truth is that most people will not face severe memory loss unless they have a serious illness such as
Alzheimer's disease. But as we age, almost every adult is faced
with memory changes that can be frustrating and unnerv-
ing. It's very common to hear people, often starting in their
forties, complain about forgetting names, forgetting what they
read, misplacing things, or forgetting to do something important. (Just yesterday, one of the authors of this book forgot an
appointment.)

Researchers have extensively studied how memory changes
with normal aging. Let's look at what they tell us about what
happens to the components of the memory process over time.
As we recall from chapter 2, the memory process can be divided into three components: sensory input, working memory,
and long-term memory.

Sensory input exhibits little change as people grow older.
Unless there is significant vision or hearing loss, people can

register information through their senses in the same way they did when they were younger. For example, Mary can scan the skeins of yarn in a knitting store to select the color she wants for an afghan. She can smell a melon to see whether it is ripe. Max can look through the selection of plants before choosing one for his garden. He can see and hear the birds in the backyard.

Working memory—the amount of information you can pay attention to at any given moment—is much the same in older and younger people. Mary can think about how much yarn she needs and what color would suit her granddaughter. She can decide which melon to buy for the neighborhood potluck. Before making his selection, Max can think about the design of his garden and the amount of direct sunlight a plant requires. He can recognize a familiar birdcall.

Long-term memory, information stored in the memory bank, is the component of memory most affected by age. The changes in long-term memory involve the ability to store and retrieve information efficiently.

As you recall from chapter 3, the process of storing information in long-term memory is called "encoding." The following common complaints demonstrate failures to encode information well enough:

- I can't keep track of where I put my glasses.
- I forget what I was planning to buy at the grocery store.
- After I've looked in all of my pockets and checked the car for my cell phone so I can plug it in at night, I find it charging in its usual place, right where I plugged it in an hour ago.
- I can't remember how to reset the digital clock in my car.

Another problem with long-term memory involves recall. You've already learned that retrieval can occur by recognition (the perception of information presented to you as something you already know) or by recall (a self-initiated search for information from long-term memory). The good news is that most people do not have problems with recognition: they say, "I know it when I see it" or "I know it when I hear it." In tests that measure recognition of words, older people do as well as or better than younger people. Retrieving information on demand (recall), however, often becomes more difficult as we grow older

Here are some examples of problems with recall:

- I have trouble coming up with names of people I know when I meet them unexpectedly.
- I can't remember the name of my medicine when someone asks me what I take.
- I don't remember to turn the ringer back on my cell phone after leaving the movie theater.
- I forgot to water my neighbor's plants when she went on vacation.

There is another aspect of memory that is so automatic we take it for granted. It's called "muscle memory." Tasks that you do repeatedly—such as driving a car, typing on a keyboard, taking a shower, washing the dishes, or tying a shoe—can all be done without conscious thought because of muscle memory. Your muscles remember how to do the task. This type of memory endures throughout life with very little change.

One more piece of good news: people gain knowledge and wisdom with age. Knowledge is defined as a pool of information acquired over a lifetime from both educational and everyday experiences. In tests that measure knowledge, older adults do as well as or better than younger people. Even though it takes greater effort to learn something new, older adults have the experience to determine what new information is important to them.

Wisdom is the ability to see the big picture, to recognize and understand the major themes of life. Through living we gain an understanding of human nature; we become more emotionally resilient; we develop an ability to learn from our many experiences, and we are able to remain more positive in the face of emotional challenges. Memory and experience allow us to recognize patterns and predict outcomes. Through living we learn to adapt to changes and see the truth as having many perspectives.

So, back to the problematic changes in memory discussed above. In chapters 7 and 8 we'll explore why encoding and recall become more difficult as we grow older.

7

Problems with Encoding

Our memories are card indexes consulted, and then put back in disorder by authorities whom we do not control.

—Cyril Connolly

It Becomes More Difficult to Pay Attention to More Than One Thing at a Time.

As you age, you may find it harder to attend to two competing activities, thoughts, or conversations. Keep in mind that the amount of information that can be held in working memory is quite limited, so what you are thinking of can be displaced even by your own new thought. External distractions such as a radio playing, someone talking, or a doorbell ringing may disrupt your concentration more now than they once did. The following examples present some common situations and potential solutions.

EXAMPLES

You are in the middle of a discussion at a party when you hear your name mentioned in a nearby conversation. This

39

momentary distraction makes you lose track of what you are saying. You may feel embarrassed and blame your failing memory, but what has actually occurred is that one thought has displaced another in your working memory. This is a common experience, and you can simply say, "Where was I? I lost my train of thought."

You have several questions to ask your doctor. When she enters the exam room, you have them well in mind. Then she starts asking you about your health. You find that you no longer remember your questions. Remembering what you intend to ask your doctor at the same time that you are answering her questions involves a division of attention. If you go to your doctor with a written list of questions, you will not have to rely on your memory.

You are in the middle of brewing coffee when the thought of an old friend comes to mind. You daydream for a moment about the last time you were skiing together in Vermont. When you leave the ski slope in your mind, you realize you're not sure how many tablespoons of coffee you have measured. If you count aloud while measuring, you will not get distracted from your task.

You are listening to the baseball game on the radio, eager to catch the score at the end of the inning. At the same time, you are sorting the mail. It seems reasonable to do these two things at once, but you suddenly realize the inning is over and you missed hearing the score. In the future, focus your attention on the game until the score is announced and then finish sorting the mail.

✳ EXERCISE: DIVIDED ATTENTION

Can you add this column of figures while you recite the names of the months of the year?

$$4$$
$$8$$
$$5$$
$$7$$
$$\underline{9}$$

This exercise demonstrates how difficult it is to pay attention to two fairly simple tasks at one time.   ✳

✳ ASSIGNMENT

During the next few days, notice if your attention is divided while you are trying to read the evening paper or listen to the news. Perhaps the phone rings or you jump up to stir the soup. Maybe someone asks you a question. Think about whether these distractions affect your ability to remember what you are reading or listening to. Are you having a problem with your memory, or are you trying to attend to too many things at once?   ✳

It Takes Greater Effort to Learn Something New.

Too many people believe the myth that "you can't teach an old dog new tricks." However, unless there is impairment of the brain, people can continue to learn and remember throughout life. Researchers have found that older adults do need to exert greater effort to learn new information than they required in the past. The term "greater effort" means different things to different people. You will need to decide whether a task is worth the effort required. Read the following examples and see if you think the tasks are worth the effort.

EXAMPLE

Mariko may want to memorize the phone numbers of her four brothers and sisters and is willing to make the necessary effort. She looks at the numbers for patterns and similarities. Some are easier than others to learn. She spends a total of an hour over the course of a week and learns them well. To keep them in her memory, she reviews them periodically. Suzanne may have the same goal of memorizing several phone numbers. After spending ten minutes trying, she thinks, "This isn't worth the effort. I can always look them up when I need them."

(For many people, learning phone numbers is no longer a priority, because they rely on the contacts stored in their cell phones. But, to some of us, knowing phone numbers of close family and friends can be comforting.)

If you decide that it is important for you to remember some new information, you must focus your attention on the task and find some means of encoding the information. As you recall from chapter 3, encoding may include paying attention to something, analyzing it, associating it with something already known, and elaborating on the details.

EXAMPLE

Your city council has just enacted new regulations regarding the collection of recycled plastic. They will now accept certain plastic containers at curbside, while others are unacceptable. You regularly use detergent, bleach, milk, cottage cheese, and yogurt containers and would like to recycle them. You decide that you want to easily remember which items to recycle without looking up the regulations or asking your neighbor each time.

The first step in learning this new information is giving your undivided attention to reading the information leaflet from the recycling center. You focus on the portion that describes what to do with plastics. The next step is thinking about how you can remember which of your commonly collected plastic items can go in the recycling bin. You note that the milk, bleach, and detergent containers are acceptable, whereas the cottage cheese and yogurt containers are not. After analyzing the situation, you realize that the three acceptable plastic items all contain liquids, whereas the others contain solids. Grouping these containers into other classifications, such as color, size, or shape, might also produce a solution to your problem.

You could easily have said, "It's too complicated for me. I can't remember all these distinctions." Instead you decided that it was important to learn, and you found a means of encoding the information. (We've noticed that the guidelines vary greatly from city to city, making compliance even more difficult!)

EXAMPLE

Yvonne has two coworkers, Ann Smith and Anne (with an "e" at the end) Miller, whose e-mail addresses start with asmith and amiller. When Yvonne wants to use one of their names in the body of an e-mail message, she puzzles over which spelling she should use. "There must be a way to remember who is who." She looks up the names in the company directory, thinks about each person's characteristics, and recognizes that Anne Miller has more energy than Ann Smith. She thinks, "E stands for energy! So it's energetic Anne Miller."

Yvonne paid attention to the spelling of the names; she figured out a way to create an association between the spellings and the persons; she repeated the association aloud. All of these efforts resulted in deeply encoding the spelling of the names.

✳ EXERCISE: LEARNING NEW INFORMATION

Here is some new information for you to learn and remember. Give it your undivided attention, and see how much effort it requires for you to answer the questions that follow the reading. The challenge is to find a way to remember the material, even if the particular subject does not interest you, and it takes greater effort to remember than you thought it would.

Cognitive Behavioral Therapy (CBT) is a brief form of psychotherapy used in the treatment of mood problems, such as depression or anxiety. CBT helps people to

1. Identify and correct inaccurate thoughts associated with depressed or anxious feelings,
2. Engage more often in enjoyable activities, and
3. Improve problem-solving skills.

The first step involves being aware of and correcting errors in thinking that are associated with problems in mood. For example, people with depression or anxiety often have distorted thoughts about themselves ("I am worthless" or "I can't do things as well as others"), their environments ("No one cares about me" or "My life is a mess"), or their futures ("I have nothing to look forward to" or "Something bad is going to happen to me"). In addition to thinking inaccurate thoughts, people with mood problems typically cut back on enjoyable activities, because they think that such activities will not be worth the effort. For example, they may stop going to neighborhood gatherings or reading the newspaper. Unfortunately, this withdrawal usually results in a vicious cycle where depressed or anxious mood leads to less activity, which in turn results in further mood problems. The second step of CBT seeks to remedy this downward spiral by increasing rewarding activity.

The third step of CBT provides instruction and guidance in specific strategies for solving problems (for example, breaking problems down into small steps). If a person wanted to meet new people, perhaps the first step might be to look into volunteer opportunities.

Now, can you answer these questions about this new information?

1. Who could benefit from cognitive behavioral therapy?
2. What is an example of a distorted thought?
3. If people are depressed, are they more or less likely to be active?
4. What is one strategy for solving problems?

See page 150 for answers.   ✳

8
Problems with Recall

A safe but sometimes chilly way of recalling the past is to force open a crammed drawer. If you are searching for anything in particular you don't find it, but something falls out at the back that is often more interesting.

—*J. M. Barrie*

It Is Increasingly Difficult to Access Familiar Names and Vocabulary Words on Demand.

Everyone knows the experience of being halted in midsentence when a word or name you need eludes you. The feeling of the word being on the tip of your tongue occurs more frequently as we age. The frustration of this experience can make us feel anxious, and this anxiety further blocks the recall process. Have you experienced anything similar to the following examples?

EXAMPLES

You began to tell a friend about the movie you saw last night, and you were flustered to discover that the title had escaped you. The more bothered you became, the further away the title seemed. Instead of giving yourself time and cues to retrieve the name of the movie from long-term memory, you found your attention focused on the frustration of forgetting.

You are discussing your college-age grandchildren with your brother. He asks what your grandson Robert is studying. You know what the subject matter is, and you know it starts with P. You are embarrassed that you can't come up with "philosophy" and can only think of the word "psychology." It is a fairly common phenomenon when a similar word interferes with your ability to find the word you want.

The next time you find yourself searching for a needed name or word try to relax, take a deep breath and see whether you can access the information by thinking of related items. If you are still unable to retrieve that word, don't fret. Often something in your conversation or environment will serve as a cue to call up the desired information.

It Takes Longer to Recall Information from Long-Term Memory.

Studies have shown that older adults take more time than younger people to recall needed information from long-term memory. When older adults are given increased time to complete a test, their performances greatly improve. Keep this in mind when you are impatient with yourself because you don't recall something immediately. As in the following example, give yourself a little more time, and see if you can come up with the information you want.

EXAMPLE

Carol was talking to her daughter-in-law, Mollie, on the telephone. Mollie asked, "What did you do over the weekend?" Carol hesitated and then responded, "Well, I guess . . . nothing." Several seconds later, she exclaimed, "Oh, I remember! We went out to dinner on Saturday night. I just couldn't think of it for a minute." This information was clearly not forgotten; it just took Carol a little time to retrieve it from long-term memory.

Expertise and familiarity in a specific area often more than compensate for the slowing down of recall. For example, a seventy-year-old crossword-puzzle buff, who spends some time every day doing crossword puzzles, may be able to recall words for commonly used clues as quickly as or more quickly than most younger people would.

✳ EXERCISE: HOW MEMORY CHANGES

True/False. Circle the answer.

T   F   1. The feeling of the word being on the tip of the tongue occurs more frequently as we age.

T   F   2. If you have always been able to do several things at once, age won't affect this ability.

T   F   3. Sensory input and working memory show little change as people grow older.

T   F   4. Older adults take longer to recall information from long-term memory.

T   F   5. People find recall more difficult than recognition.

T   F   6. One way to access well-known information when you can't recall it is to provide yourself with cues by thinking of related items.

See page 150 for answers.   ✳

Part III

Factors
That Affect
Memory

9

You and Your Memory
A Self-inventory

EXAMPLE

Pauline recently moved from Collinsville, Illinois, her lifelong hometown, to an apartment building near her son's home in Chicago. She had mixed feelings about moving. In Collinsville she had many friends and volunteered every week at the high school. She regularly attended an exercise class and often went out for lunch after church with the same group of people. After her husband died, however, she decided it would be best to move nearer to her son and his family. The move was stressful, because she had to reduce the belongings of a family home to fit the space of a two-bedroom apartment. She spent many weeks making decisions about what to take and how to get rid of unwanted items. By the time she arrived in her new apartment, she was too exhausted to organize things well. She missed her friends at home and found it hard to meet new people and get involved in activities. She felt sad and somewhat hopeless about creating a satisfying new life in Chicago.

For the first time, Pauline began to question her memory. She couldn't find her address book in her new apartment. She got lost driving home from the library. She fell asleep after putting some potatoes on to boil and woke up to the smell of a burned pan. She said to herself, "What is happening to me? Maybe I'm getting Alzheimer's disease."

Pauline made an appointment with a geriatrician and told him her fears about her memory. Dr. Sloan reviewed her recent history and did some tests to rule out physical causes for her forgetting. He reported that the test results were normal and that he believed the many changes brought about by her move had temporarily affected her memory.

Certain factors can affect memory for people of all ages. The effect of these factors is likely to be greater as we age, because older people often experience more of these negative influences at the same time. The following factors commonly affect memory:

Effort and attitude
    Problems with attention
    Negative expectations
    Inactivity
    Lack of organization in daily life
Problems with mood
    Depression
    Loss and grief
    Anxiety
    Stress
Health issues
    Some physical illnesses
    Some medications
    Vision and hearing problems
    Fatigue
    Alcohol
    Poor nutrition

As you read through the next three chapters, think about which of these factors might be affecting your memory. If you are aware of possible causes of memory problems, you are more likely to find solutions.

10

Check Your Effort
and Attitude

I have the most ill-regulated memory. It does those things which it ought not to do and leaves undone the things it ought to have done. But it has not yet gone on strike altogether.

—Dorothy L. Sayers

The four factors discussed in this chapter are problems with attention, negative expectations, inactivity, and lack of organization. Are any of these factors creating problems for you? Do you recognize yourself in any of the examples in this chapter?

Problems with Attention

Inadequate Attention

In the discussion of encoding in chapter 3, we emphasized the importance of focusing attention on what you want to remember. If you really want to remember something, paying adequate attention is the first step. In the following examples, not paying adequate attention affected how well new information was encoded.

EXAMPLES

A new resident of Brad's apartment building, Lia Blair, meets him at the mailboxes and introduces herself. He greets her by name and begins a friendly conversation. When they are joined by another resident a few minutes later, Brad discovers that he cannot recall Lia's name.

Ramona bought some expensive concert tickets and made a mental note to take them out of her purse when she got home and put them in a special place so she could easily find them later. The next morning, as Ramona got in her car to leave for work, she realized she hadn't put the tickets safely away, nor could she find the tickets in her purse. She went back to her apartment and found them on the nightstand. She was relieved to know that the tickets weren't lost, but she couldn't understand why she had no recollection of having put them on the nightstand.

Juan's neighbor asks him to feed her cat while she is gone over the weekend. She tells him where the cat food is kept, how much and how often to feed her, and where she hides the spare key. When Juan goes to feed the cat, he is horrified to discover that he does not recall where the key is hidden. Because he is unfamiliar with cats, he paid close attention to the instructions regarding feeding, but he assumed that he would remember where the key was hidden and did not pay attention to that detail.

All of these examples illustrate problems in encoding. Brad heard and spoke Lia Blair's name but didn't encode the information into long-term memory for recollection. Ramona absentmindedly took the tickets from her purse and placed them on the nightstand. She had not paid adequate attention to what she was doing. Juan was so concerned about providing good care for the cat that he paid attention only to the information about food.

Paying adequate attention to details can eliminate some instances of forgetting. Ask yourself, "When is it really important for me to pay attention?" At these times, put some effort into focusing your awareness on the task or information at hand.

Distractions

Being distracted poses another potential problem with attention. Because the amount of information that can be held in your working memory is limited, any sound, sight, or thought may distract you and displace what is currently in your working memory. You are certain to have had one or more of the following experiences.

EXAMPLES

You go into the kitchen to get the scissors and forget what you went for. Perhaps, on your way, you wondered whether the mail had come. This new thought replaced the thought of the scissors you needed from the kitchen.

You may leave your umbrella in the doctor's office because you are thinking about getting your prescription filled before the pharmacy closes. (Have you noticed that if you get outside and it's raining, you remember you forgot your umbrella and go back inside to retrieve it?)

You're driving to a movie with a friend. Her conversation draws your attention away from noticing exactly where you are, and you forget to get into the left-turn lane until it's too late.

These experiences are familiar to people of all ages, but as we grow older, we do find it more difficult to pay attention to more than one thing at a time. Rather than thinking that you can do nothing about these frustrating experiences, try to recognize the limitations of working memory and cut out distractions when possible. It is especially important to give your undivided attention to situations that could be potentially dangerous, such as driving, cooking, and taking medications. For example, when you are driving in an unfamiliar place or you need to change driving lanes in traffic, you may want to ask your passenger to stop talking temporarily.

✳ EXERCISE: DISTRACTIONS

Below are two short stories. Read the first one in a quiet room, and then read the second one with some competition for your attention, such as the TV or radio.

First Story
Nina had three tickets to a country music festival. She invited her cousin and her best friend. She packed a picnic lunch of sandwiches, potato salad, and fruit. They put their plaid blanket under a tree. The vocals were split between the guitarist and the drummer. The concert ended at midnight after three encores.

See how many details you can recall from this story. Now remember to turn on the radio or TV.

Second Story
A lifeguard at a rocky beach came to work on his silver motorcycle. He changed from blue jeans to a bathing suit

and put his whistle around his neck. He hollered at three teenagers, who were out too far, to come closer to shore. At sunset, his blonde girlfriend brought him a hot dog, a Coke, and some potato chips.

Did you notice differences in your ability to remember the details in these two stories?   ✳

Negative Expectations

Compared with younger people, older adults may be less optimistic about their ability to remember. They often say, "I just can't remember anything anymore," whereas younger people blame forgetting on a lack of effort or interest. When we expect that we are going to fail at something, that expectation is likely to increase the possibility of failure. Negative attitudes about memory often cause us to

- Put less effort into remembering
- Avoid tasks that require memory
- Feel anxious when our memories are tested in daily life

EXAMPLE

Julie attended a volunteer appreciation banquet. Although she recognized many faces, she felt embarrassed and anxious when she could not address people by name. She thought, "I can't remember names anymore!" Since that time she has avoided gatherings if she doesn't know everyone who will be there. Although her son-in-law gave her a book on how to remember names, she is sure that those techniques will not be useful.

When you are faced with a task of memory, do you find yourself saying, "I'll never be able to do this. What's the use of trying?" Sometimes we give ourselves negative messages without being aware of it. Be conscious of your self-defeating thoughts about your ability to remember. Substitute this thought: "I'm not sure this will work, but I'll give it a good try."

Inactivity

We frequently read that mental, social, and physical activity is good for the mind and body. As you read this section, think about whether increased activity might benefit your memory. Examine your attitude and effort to see whether your outlook is affecting your level of activity.

Lack of Mental Stimulation

The old adage "use it or lose it" is often applied to memory functioning. Keeping mentally active and using memory skills may enhance your ability to remember. Here are some examples of mental stimulation:

- Attending an adult education class
- Participating in a discussion group
- Doing crossword puzzles
- Playing cards or board games
- Practicing online memory games
- Answering *Jeopardy* or other quiz show questions
- Learning to use the features on an electronic device
- Reading a challenging book
- Using newly learned memory techniques

EXAMPLE

Karen has always had a great interest in current events. Although she reads the newspaper daily, she has lately found it difficult to retain the information she needs in order to determine her position on political issues. Rather than give up, she joins the current events discussion group at the library. She enjoys the lively discussions and finds that her memory for issues is reinforced by preparing for the group and hearing what others think about them.

Lack of Social Interaction

Many experts agree that social involvement is a major factor in maintaining or improving mental capacities. When days are uncommitted and unstructured, there is less incentive to focus and organize your thoughts and less need to remember. In social contact you have the opportunity to talk about the events of your life, which reinforces the memory of what you have done and learned.

EXAMPLES

You receive an e-mail from your sister telling you that your niece has made an offer on her first home. When your sister calls later in the week and says, "Jenny got it!," you have no idea what she is talking about. Before you assume that your memory is failing, consider the fact that you saw very few people over the week and told no one about the news. If you tell a friend about any new information you receive, you encode it more deeply and greatly increase your chances of remembering it.

Dan lives alone with no relatives nearby. He suffers from severe arthritis and heart problems. He is uncomfortable and fearful when away from home. His neighbor stops for a brief visit when he brings in his mail each day and notices that Dan is becoming more forgetful. Dan rarely knows what day it is and tells his neighbor that he has forgotten his last two doctors' appointments. When he finally sees the doctor, Dan has an ulcer on his foot that needs attention. The doctor orders a visiting nurse to treat the wound and a home health aide three times a week to provide personal care and homemaking services. After a few weeks, Dan's neighbor notices that Dan seems more alert and always remembers what day it is, since he looks forward to the aide, Hilary, coming on Monday, Wednesday, and Friday. Dan told his neighbor, "I like to keep up with the news now because Hilary is really interested in the election and always wants to hear my opinion."

Lack of Physical Activity

Exercise has many known benefits. We know that exercise strengthens bones and muscles and reduces the risk of cardiovascular disease, diabetes, and stress. Study after study also show that increased fitness levels result in improvement on cognitive tests. In animal studies, brain scans show the birth of new neurons in mice who exercise; brain scans of mice that do not exercise do not show these new neurons. Studies have also shown that exercising several times a week for thirty to sixty minutes may result in an increase in brain volume and improved memory and thinking. Although researchers are still investigating how much exercise is needed for maximum benefit, all researchers recommend weekly aerobic exercise for positive cognitive results.

EXAMPLE

Kate has cut back on physical exercise due to her busy schedule and the severe winter weather in Minnesota. In addition to feeling less fit, she has noticed more memory lapses. Friends have been trying to get her to go to an exercise class, but she just hasn't felt like it. She finally gives in and goes to an aerobics class. She finds it difficult for the first couple of weeks, but since she has paid for an eight-week class, she sticks with it. After about a month, Kate notices that she has more energy and that her mind seems a bit sharper. She reads an article in the paper about the relationship between physical exercise and mental functioning. She thanks her friend and says, "Maybe this class will be good for my mind as well as my body."

Lack of Organization in Daily Life

Many instances of forgetting and losing things can be traced to a disorganized lifestyle. When you don't have a systematic way of keeping track of your appointments, returning things to their correct places in your home, paying bills, or storing important papers in a safe place, you are more likely to be forgetful. Many people have developed a lifelong habit of being organized, while others are disorganized and have never been bothered by it. If you think that some of your instances of forgetting are due to a lack of organization, you may want to develop some new organizational habits. It does take work to make changes, but organization saves effort in the long run.

EXAMPLES

Cathy complained, "I always write things down. I know about keeping lists, but then I can't find the lists." At a memory course at her recreation center, she heard other participants describe the same situation. The teacher advised them to keep all lists of things to buy or do in one convenient place. Cathy realized she had been making lists on odd scraps of paper and leaving them all over the house. She remedied the situation by keeping a notebook for lists on her kitchen table.

You notice that your credit card bill is unusually large. You're positive that you paid last month's bill, but, when you look at your bank statement, there is no record of payment. You search for the bill in all the likely places with no success. After you've called the credit card company to complain, you discover last month's bill in a book you're reading. No wonder you forgot to pay it! Most people can't keep track of household finances without some organized system. When your bills are scattered throughout the house and you have no regular schedule for paying them, it's very easy to neglect one. (To avoid penalties, some people set up their accounts so their bills are paid automatically online every month.)

✳ ASSIGNMENT

Choose **one** area of your life in which you think getting organized will help you remember:

_____ Keeping track of my purse/keys/glasses/other

_____ Remembering when I last gave to my favorite charity

_____ Sending birthday cards to family and friends on time

_____ Paying my bills when they're due

_____ Keeping track of the scissors/tape/pencil sharpener/wrapping paper/other

_____ Putting gas in the car before it's nearly empty

_____ Taking the garbage out

_____ Your choice _____

Now that you have chosen one, think of a way to organize this area of your life so you will remember. For example, you might put up a hook where you will **always** hang your keys.

The problem:

_____

_____

_____

Your solution:

_____

_____

_____

The results:

_____

_____

_____

After you have accomplished this goal, why not choose another?

The problem:

_____

_____

_____

Your solution:

_____

_____

_____

The results:

_____

_____

_____ ✳

11

Could Your Mood
Be the Problem?

Memories are contrary things; if you quit chasing
them and turn your back, they often return on
their own.

—Stephen King

You may be surprised to learn that your mood can affect your
memory. If you are experiencing depression, grief, anxiety, or
stress, you may not recognize the symptoms or realize that
these conditions can create problems with memory. We hope
this chapter and its examples will help you evaluate your mood
and its effect on your memory.

Depression

Many people believe that depression is a normal part of
aging, but depression is an illness—a treatable illness. We
know that memory problems often accompany depression
and that, if the depression is treated, the memory problems
improve. The National Institute of Mental Health website
(www.nimh.nih.gov/health) lists the following symptoms of
depression:

- Persistent sad, anxious, or "empty" feelings
- Feelings of hopelessness or pessimism
- Feelings of guilt, worthlessness, or helplessness
- Irritability, restlessness
- Loss of interest in activities or hobbies once pleasurable, including sex
- Fatigue and decreased energy
- Difficulty concentrating, remembering details, and making decisions
- Insomnia, early-morning wakefulness, or excessive sleeping
- Overeating or appetite loss
- Thoughts of suicide, suicide attempts
- Aches or pains, headaches, cramps, or digestive problems that do not ease even with treatment

How Does Depression Affect Memory?

Motivation: When you are depressed you don't care about remembering your new neighbor's name, the time of your exercise class, or who's running for city council. None of these things seems important.

Concentration: Even if you want to read the book for the next book club meeting, depression can make you feel foggy and not able to focus on the task.

Perception: If you are depressed you may view a few instances of forgetting as a sign that you can't remember anything at all.

EXAMPLE

Ed has experienced episodes of depression for several years. His friends and family had noticed that, when he was feeling depressed, he forgot appointments, confused the names of his neighbors, and couldn't remember what happened the day before. The first few times this occurred, his family wondered if he was getting Alzheimer's disease. The family encouraged Ed to see his physician. After a full evaluation Dr. Garcia concluded that Ed's memory problems might improve if his depression was treated by a combination of medication and counseling. He also recommended that, while Ed remained depressed, his family set up his pillbox, help him with paying bills, and remind him of appointments.

Loss and Grief

When we have experienced a significant loss, we are often overwhelmed with feelings of pain and sadness. It is difficult to focus on anything outside ourselves, and it is harder to concentrate. Memory problems frequently accompany grief and will decrease over time unless the person who is mourning develops depression.

Most people think primarily of death when we talk about loss and grief. In fact, a feeling of loss may accompany many different experiences, including a move, major surgery, retirement, vision or hearing problems, illness of a friend or family member, changes in financial circumstances, death of a pet, marriage of a child or friend, and changes in health. Even a change you choose to make, such as retiring or moving, can be accompanied by a feeling of loss. When two or more of these experiences occur at once, the effect is greatly increased.

EXAMPLES

Sean had been ready to retire for several years when the day finally arrived. He looked forward to sleeping late, having no boss to answer to, and spending time in his basement workshop. He was surprised to discover, however, that he often felt sad and at loose ends. He also noticed that he was forgetting things. With his wife's encouragement, he volunteered to deliver Meals on Wheels to shut-ins and began a drawing class. As he felt more useful, his sadness diminished, along with much of his forgetfulness.

Jeff had been dating Kristin for a year and a half. He thought things were going well and planned on a future with her. After the holidays, Kristin told him that she hadn't been happy in their relationship for a while and that she wanted to stop seeing him. Jeff initially was very angry and told himself he was better off without her. As days passed, he found himself tearful and overwhelmed. He couldn't pay attention to his work and forgot his friend's birthday party. He felt like his mind was deteriorating. He wondered whether he was losing his memory, and he didn't know what to do about it. After several months passed, he realized that he was feeling better and that his memory was better, too. With the lessening of Jeff's grief, his memory returned to normal.

Anxiety

Anxiety is characterized as inner distress accompanied by physical symptoms and vague fears. Many people who are highly anxious are unable to focus on anything outside of themselves. Their minds are so filled with worries that they cannot pay attention to external happenings, and their memory failures affect their daily functioning.

Some symptoms of anxiety are

- Nervousness, worry, or fear
- Apprehension or a sense of imminent doom
- Panic spells
- Difficulty concentrating
- Insomnia

- Fear of potential physical illnesses
- Heart pounding or racing
- Upset stomach or diarrhea
- Sweating
- Dizziness or light-headedness
- Restlessness or jumpiness
- Irritability

EXAMPLE

Diane describes herself as someone who has always been a worrier, but it has gotten worse as she has grown older. She worries about her unmarried son, her granddaughter's thumb-sucking, her own high blood pressure, and her arthritis, which could affect her ability to take care of her home. She feels agitated, doesn't sleep well, spends most of the day worrying, and is unable to remember things very well.

When she is in the clinic to get a blood pressure reading, Diane mentions her anxiety to the nurse, who suggests that she should discuss it with the doctor. Dr. Hall recommends a cognitive behavioral therapy group for people who are anxious or depressed, where Diane might learn new ways of dealing with her anxiety and benefit from the group support. In the group, Diane recognizes that she has no control over her son's unmarried state and her granddaughter's thumb-sucking. She vows to try to take them off her worry list. The group helps her consider options for the future in case she is unable to take care of her home.

Diane knows that she will continue to be a worrier; however, when she reminds herself of the uselessness of worrying about those things that she cannot control, some of her symptoms of anxiety are alleviated, including memory problems. As she worries less, she finds she can concentrate and remember better.

Stress

When we are feeling stressed, pressured, or rushed, it is often impossible to

- Pay adequate attention to learning new information
- Concentrate on the details we want to recall
- Relax long enough to let a memory surface

We are more likely to forget things when we are under major stress—due to factors such as moving, illness, loss, or retirement—or even when we are under minor stress caused by experiences such as being late to an appointment, misplacing the house keys, preparing for company, or getting ready for a trip. It is important to realize that we may forget more frequently at times like these and that memory usually improves as the stress is reduced.

EXAMPLE

You have been extremely busy all week getting ready for a visit from your son and his family, who live in California. The sink becomes clogged, and the plumber is available only during the time when you are picking up the family from the airport. You ask your neighbor if you can give her a house key when you leave for the airport, so she can let the plumber in. To your horror, you forget to leave the key. Because you were stressed, overloaded, and rushing, you forgot to do what you wanted to do most. In a case like this, it's best to take action the moment you think of it.

12

Ask Your Doctor about Health Issues

God gave us memory so that we might have roses in December.

—*J. M. Barrie*

EXAMPLE

Ellen's son is very concerned about her forgetfulness. He continually tells her that she should try harder and feels that she should learn some new memory techniques. He learns about a memory course from a neighbor and insists that his mother take the course, although she is not enthusiastic. He calls the instructor to enroll his mother in the class and describes her problems. She repeats herself frequently and sometimes forgets that he has called. She is having trouble keeping track of her bills and has dropped out of her card-playing group. As he paints the picture of his mother's memory problems and expresses his conviction that she could remember if she really tried, the instructor wonders whether Ellen's memory problems may be related to a health issue. She suggests to the son that he should go with his mother to her next medical appointment and discuss his concerns with her doctor.

Physical health and mental functioning are very closely linked. Factors such as physical illnesses, medications, vision and hearing problems, fatigue, alcohol, and nutrition may affect your memory. Ask your doctor whether your memory changes may be related to a health problem or medication.

Some Physical Illnesses

Even though many older people do not develop severe memory loss, memory problems can be a sign that the body is not functioning properly. Some physical illnesses can aggravate an already existing mild memory problem, or they can cause memory changes in a person who has not previously experienced memory loss.

On the one hand, conditions such as infection, fever, dehydration, and thyroid problems can cause temporary changes in memory that improve when the condition is treated. Urinary tract infections are notorious for causing memory problems and confusion in older people.

On the other hand, some types of diseases or injuries that cause damage to the brain may not be reversible. Alzheimer's disease is the most common cause of irreversible memory loss. (For more information on Alzheimer's disease and other causes of dementia, see the appendix.)

Strokes and traumatic injury to the head often cause memory problems that show improvement in the months after the trauma but frequently leave some irreversible changes.

If you are concerned about your memory and want to rule out a physical cause, the first step is to see your doctor, who is familiar with your medical history. Some physicians receive little training in assessing the mental status of older people. In that case it may be worthwhile to consult a physician with specific training in geriatrics or neurology, who has the diagnostic skills to distinguish among a wide assortment of possible causes of memory loss. A medical assessment often includes

- A social and medical history taken from both the patient and a relative or friend
- A thorough physical exam
- A neuropsychological exam, which is a series of tests that provides information about the thought processes
- Blood tests, which are used to detect thyroid, kidney, and liver malfunctions; certain nutritional deficiencies, such as pernicious anemia or vitamin B_{12} deficiency; infections; and metabolic and chemical imbalances
- Urinalysis, which is used to detect infections in the urinary tract

Other tests that may be indicated include

- A CT scan of the brain (computerized axial tomogram), which is a diagnostic imaging procedure that uses a combination of x-rays and computer technology to produce horizontal images (often called slices) of the brain
- An MRI of the brain (magnetic resonance imaging), which is a diagnostic procedure that uses a combination of large magnets, radiofrequencies, and a computer to produce detailed images of organs and structures within the body, including the brain
- A PET scan of the brain (positron emission tomogram), which is a nuclear medicine scan that shows how the brain and its tissues are working (Other imaging tests, such as MRI and CT scans, only reveal the structure of the brain.)
- An EEG (electroencephalogram), which is a measurement of electrical activity (brain waves) in the brain

- A lumbar puncture (spinal tap), which is an analysis of spinal fluid that can detect malignancies, neurosyphilis, and certain infections

EXAMPLE

When Meg, the housecleaner, arrived at Theresa's apartment for her weekly visit, she found Theresa in bed and quite confused. When Meg asked Theresa whether she had had breakfast, Theresa said she wasn't sure. Also, she could not remember Meg's name or exactly why Meg was there. Since Theresa had never been confused in the past, Meg consulted with a neighbor, who agreed that Theresa should go to the emergency room. The physicians at the hospital discovered that she had a serious urinary tract infection and admitted her to the hospital. When Theresa's infection cleared up, her confusion disappeared, and she returned home feeling mentally and physically well.

Some Medications

Prescription and over-the-counter medications can affect your memory, because they can slow your thinking and make you feel drowsy or foggy. They can diminish your attention or concentration, making it harder to register information in your working memory.

Most, but not all, of the time, memory is affected within days after starting a new medication or increasing the dose. Sometimes the change is noticed by the person taking the medication, and sometimes the change is more noticeable to other people. A memory problem due to medication is seldom permanent, however. In fact, the problem may go away on its own as you continue to take the medicine and your body adjusts to it. If the problem doesn't go away, talk with your doctors to find out if there are other medications you can take instead.

No one can tell who will have a memory problem from a medication, and it can happen to anyone. Some things, however, make a person more likely to have memory problems with medications:

- Side effects from medications in the past
- Low weight
- Older age
- A sudden change in health
- Taking several other medications
- Taking more (or less) of a medication than you are supposed to
- Taking a medication in combination with alcohol
- A medical condition like Alzheimer's disease that is already affecting memory
- Some kinds of liver disease
- Heart failure
- Kidney failure

Although some medications affect memory and attention more than others do, the same medications don't cause the same problems in everyone. Medications that have a higher risk of memory problems include

- Prescription sleeping or anxiety medications
    Ambien (zolpidem)
    Ativan (lorazepam)
    Lunesta (eszopiclone)
    Sonata (zaleplon)

Valium (diazepam)
Xanax (alprazolam)
- Urinary incontinence medications
  Detrol (tolterodine)
  Ditropan or Oxytrol (oxybutynin)
  Enablex (darifenacin)
  Sanctura (trospium)
  Toviaz (fesoterodine)
  Vesicare (solifenacin)
- Muscle relaxants
  Lioresal (baclofen)
  Flexeril (cyclobenzaprine)
  Skelaxin (metaxalone)
  Soma (carisoprodol)
- Neurontin (gabapentin)
- Over-the-counter allergy or sleeping pills
  Benadryl or Sominex (diphenhydramine)
  Chlor-Trimeton (chlorpheniramine)
  Unisom (doxylamine)
- Narcotic pain medications
  MS Contin and other brands of morphine
  Duragesic or Actiq (fentanyl)
  Oxycontin and other brands of oxycodone
  hydrocodone (found in Vicodin, Norco, Lortab and
    other brands)

The effect of "statin" cholesterol-lowering medications is unclear. When starting treatment, they might cause memory problems in some people. But if taken for a year or more, they might reduce the chance for dementia. They include

Crestor (rosuvastatin)
Lescol (fluvastatin)

Lipitor (atorvastatin)

Mevacor (lovastatin)

Pravachol (pravastatin)

Zocor (simvastatin)

Memory problems can happen at any time during treatment, but they happen more often when getting started or when increasing the dose.

Medications are only one of many causes of memory problems. If you think you are having a memory problem from a medication, you should talk to your doctors or pharmacists. **Never stop or reduce your medications on your own.** You and your doctor can together decide whether your memory problem may be due to the medication and what to do about it.

When it comes to side effects of medicines, prevention is key. You can be a partner in preventing memory problems due to medications by

- Keeping a list of medications and showing it to your doctors and pharmacists before you start or change the dose of a medicine
- Working with your doctors to try to stop medications you may no longer need
- Not drinking alcohol if you think your memory might be affected by your medications
- Talking with your doctors or pharmacists about scheduling the taking of your medications to lessen their effect on your memory
- Telling your doctors and pharmacists if you think your memory is affected by a medicine, so that they can try to prevent this problem from happening again with the same or similar medications

(This section on medications was written by Tami Remington, Pharm.D., Clinical Associate Professor, University of Michigan, Ann Arbor.)

EXAMPLE

Tom has been feeling tired and foggy, and he is forgetting more than he used to. His daughter suggests that he see his family doctor for consultation. Dr. Brown takes a complete history, including a review of medications. She discovers that Tom has begun to take over-the-counter sleeping pills to treat his insomnia, along with the blood pressure medication that she had prescribed at the last visit. Dr. Brown recognizes that the combination of the two drugs could be causing Tom's fatigue and memory problems. She prescribes a short-acting sleeping pill, so that this medication will be out of Tom's system during the daytime. Tom finds that, over time, his memory improves with this adjustment of medications.

Vision and Hearing Problems

A person with vision or hearing problems may blame his memory if he can't recall information or experiences. In fact, the problem may not be in the memory at all. When you can't see or hear clearly, the information will not be encoded correctly. It is important to admit when you can't hear adequately and ask others to speak up. If you are unable to read printed material, ask for a large-print copy or ask someone to read it to you. Get regularly scheduled vision and auditory tests to make sure that you are getting the eyeglasses and hearing aids you need. Vision and hearing abilities can change dramatically, and new technology may compensate for losses.

EXAMPLES

Your neighbor suggests that you call a Realtor whose name is Abbott. When you call the realty company, you ask for Mr. Babcock. The problem here may not be your memory; your neighbor may have mumbled, or you may have trouble hearing. If you want to remember something correctly, ask the person to repeat it, spell it, and write it down.

At the doctor's office, the receptionist gives you an insurance form to complete at home. "Sign in these three places, and mail it off," she says, pointing to three blanks. When you get home, you are confused by all the blank spaces and say, "I've already forgotten what she told me." The problem may not be in your memory. You may not have seen the spaces she pointed to. Next time, ask her to mark the spaces with a red X.

Fatigue

Fatigue affects concentration and slows down the recall process. We are more likely to have trouble learning new information, because focus and attention are impaired when we're tired. If we can figure out which times of the day we are most alert, we can do tasks that involve new learning at those times.

If insomnia is a problem for you, consider talking to your doctor about it. (A good website on sleep habits is http://healthysleep.med.harvard.edu/.)

EXAMPLES

You usually read at bedtime because it puts you to sleep. However, you can't keep the characters straight in the book you're reading, and this frustrates you. You might try reading the book when you are more alert. If you want to read before dozing off, read something you don't care about remembering.

You have just finished attending the third lecture of a six-week series on health problems at your local library. You were especially looking forward to last week's lecture on diabetes, because your husband has diabetes in his family. You realize, however, that you remember little of the material because you were especially tired that day. For the next lecture, you resolve to be rested and ready to take notes.

Alcohol

Alcohol can affect your memory in two different ways. First, many people find that they are less able to tolerate alcohol as they grow older; two drinks may have been tolerated well in the past but are now too much. As far as memory is concerned, there is a greater effect on the brain if you have four drinks in one night than if you have one drink on each of four nights. Second, long-term abuse of alcohol can cause irreversible memory loss.

In addition to the direct effects of alcohol on memory, alcohol consumption can cause or make worse other factors that affect your memory:

- **Depression**: Alcohol acts as a depressant on the central nervous system.
- **Decreased nutritional status**: Some people who drink excessively do not eat an adequate or nutritious diet.

Poor Nutrition

We read articles and see news reports all the time about foods that are thought to be beneficial or harmful for health and cognition. Some foods that have been on the "bad foods" list have been redeemed and now are recommended in moderation. Reversals like this make it very difficult to know what specific foods we should eat to help our brains be healthy, even as researchers vigorously investigate whether certain foods can improve brain function.

What we do know is that a balanced diet contributes to overall health. The best advice at this time is to eat fresh fruits and vegetables, whole-grain cereals and breads, and a variety of foods rich in protein.

13

Let's Review Again

Are you frustrated because you forgot to mail a birthday card? Are you avoiding social occasions because you don't have the energy? Did you miss an important meeting because you entered it wrong on your calendar? Are you misplacing things more often than you used to?

So far in this book we have looked at the different factors that affect memory. Now we ask you to think about which of these factors might be affecting you.

Once you have identified the factors that are affecting you, you may wish to go back and reread the information in chapters 9–12 about those factors. To address some of these factors, you may need to see a physician, counselor, or other professional for treatment. For other factors, you may find ways to make changes in your environment or lifestyle to address the problem. To get you started, part IV is full of memory improvement techniques that many people find effective.

✳ SELF-INVENTORY OF FACTORS AFFECTING MEMORY

	Never	Some-times	Always
Problems with attention	_____	_____	_____
Negative expectations	_____	_____	_____
Inactivity	_____	_____	_____
Lack of organization	_____	_____	_____
Depression	_____	_____	_____
Loss and grief	_____	_____	_____
Anxiety	_____	_____	_____
Stress	_____	_____	_____
Physical illness	_____	_____	_____
Medication	_____	_____	_____
Vision problems	_____	_____	_____
Hearing problems	_____	_____	_____
Fatigue	_____	_____	_____
Alcohol	_____	_____	_____
Nutrition	_____	_____	_____

✳

✳ EXERCISE: FACTORS THAT AFFECT MEMORY

True/False. Circle the answer.

T   F   1. Problems with vision or hearing can affect your memory.

T   F   2. Memory is not affected by mood.

T   F   3. Poor memory is often due to lack of attention.

T   F   4. Negative expectations have no effect on memory performance.

T   F   5. Lack of concentration can be a symptom of anxiety or depression.

T   F   6. Problems with your health can cause increased forgetting.

T   F   7. Medications affect everyone the same way.

T   F   8. Even if you're looking forward to moving to a new place, you may notice some memory problems after you move.

T   F   9. Once your memory begins to get worse, it will never improve.

T   F   10. Increasing activity, through mental stimulation, social interaction, or physical exercise, may benefit memory.

See page 150 for answers.   ✳

Part IV

Techniques for Improving Your Memory

14

Exploring Memory Improvement Strategies

So far we have learned about how memory works and about how memory changes as we age. We hope you have identified any factors in your life that may be affecting your memory. Now we are ready to explore strategies and techniques that can make a difference in your ability to remember.

There are several strategies for remembering different kinds of information. Once you have decided that you want to improve your memory in a particular area, you can select strategies for change. In this chapter we introduce seventeen techniques for improving your memory. In the chapters that follow we describe these techniques and how to use them.

Some techniques improve the way you encode information, so you can retrieve it more easily. They include

- Association
- Visualization
- Active observation
- Elaboration
- Repetition

Some techniques involve cues in your environment, such as notes, lists, signs, or buzzers:

- Written reminders
- Auditory reminders
- Environmental change

One technique is extremely useful for remembering whether you did what you meant to do:

- Self-instruction

Five techniques help when you have several items to remember:

- Story method
- Chunking
- First-letter cues
- Create a word
- Categorization

Some techniques are helpful in retrieving information that you know well but can't quite bring to mind:

- Cue yourself
- Alphabet search
- Review in advance

Some of these techniques will be familiar; others will seem strange. It is difficult to know which ones will be useful for you without trying them several times. Look for chances to experiment.

It can be fun and rewarding to figure out a way to remember and then to succeed. In some cases, however, you may decide that the effort needed is not worth the benefit gained. Recognize that the choice is yours to make.

Here's the best way to use these memory improvement techniques:

1. Choose something specific that you want to remember.
2. Review the possible techniques and select one.
3. Try the technique. (If it works, congratulations!)
4. If your chosen technique does not work, try something else.
5. Don't feel defeated if some things are particularly hard to remember. Ask yourself whether it really matters.

15

Improving Your Ability to Encode

Dates are hard to remember because they consist
of figures; figures are monotonously unstriking in
appearance, and they don't take hold, they form no
pictures, and so they give the eye no chance to help.
Pictures are the thing. Pictures can make dates stick.

—*Mark Twain*

The five techniques described in this chapter can be used to encode almost any kind of new information. It takes thought and practice to incorporate these techniques into everyday life but they work so well they are likely to become a habit. The examples in this chapter illustrate strategies for encoding information, and the exercises let you practice these strategies.

Association: Associate What You Want to Remember with What You Already Know.

"Association" is the process of forming mental connections between what we want to remember and what we already know. Although we form many associations automatically, we also can consciously create a connection between new information and information that we know well. By doing this, we are deliberately encoding new information. Once you make an association, you will remember it better if you repeat it several times, either in your head or out loud.

This technique can be used to remember such things as

- The name of your new neighbor
- The street where your friend lives
- The title of a movie you want to recommend
- Whether to turn right or left to get to the restaurant
- The number of the bus to catch for your friend's house

EXAMPLES

Beth: My new neighbor's name was Marsha. For some reason I had a hard time remembering her name, and I decided to use association to try to remember it. After looking carefully at Marsha, I noticed she had white, fluffy hair. I decided that I could remember her name by associating "Marsha" with "marshmallow." Each time I saw her, I associated her hair with a big marshmallow and said to myself, "Marshmallow means Marsha."

Miles: I could never remember whether my gas tank is on the right or left side of the car. Each time I went to fill up, I had to think about which way to approach the gas pumps, and I felt aggravated. I decided to consciously find an association that would register the information once and for all. I first noted that my gas cap is on the right side. What could I associate with "right"? This was easier than I thought—I have a red car! I associated the "r" in red with the "r" in right. Now when I go to the gas station, I say, "In this red car, the gas cap is on the right." Problem solved!

(You may be saying to yourself, "Sure—he happens to have a red car with the gas tank on the right. What about my car that is black with the gas tank on the right?" In this case, you may need to go beyond the obvious. You may notice that both "black" and "right" have five letters. Again, problem solved! However, if you can't find an association between your car and its gas tank, you need a different strategy. How about repeating "right is right" or "left is logical"? That should do the trick.)

✳ EXERCISE: ASSOCIATION

Create an association between the following new information and something you already know.

1. You must remember to take the entrance marked "west" on the expressway to get to the doctor's office.

_____

_____

_____

2. You want to remember the year you retired, which is 2008.

_____

_____

_____

3. You want to remember Rose Campbell's name.

_____

_____

_____

4. You want to remember the name "Turner Medical Clinic."

_____

_____

_____

See page 151 for possible answers.   ✳

Visualization: Visualize a Picture of What You Want to Remember.

It's often said that a picture is worth a thousand words. Visualization takes advantage of this concept by consciously creating an image in your mind of what you want to remember: a task, a number, a name, a word, or a thought. If you take the time to create a meaningful picture and then hold that picture in your mind for a few moments, you are more likely to remember.

This technique can be used to remember such things as

- Items you need to buy at the grocery store
- The route from the airport terminal to where you parked your car
- The laundry basket you want to bring up from the basement
- The name of a new breakfast cereal you want to try
- An icon on your computer

EXAMPLES

Sue: I love to tell my friends about my favorite restaurant. It's so expensive that I can only go there once a year, so I don't see the name very often. It's called Justine's, which is a name I have trouble remembering. However, I do know that they have a young chef, so I imagine a very youthful face with a big chef's hat on, and think, "Why, he's 'just a teen.'"

Henry: I get frustrated when I put on my coat, walk to the back of my yard to retrieve something from the garage, and then forget what I went out to get. I've learned from experience that, if I take the time to picture what I'm getting up for, I can usually remember. Yesterday I wanted the flashlight from my car. I remembered it as blue, and I envisioned myself using it to look in the attic. When I got to the car, I had no trouble remembering that I wanted my blue flashlight.

Tim: I took a memory improvement course through my local adult education department. The instructor taught us the technique of visualization and I decided to practice this technique to remember three errands. I had to go to the hardware store to buy a rake, to the jeweler to have my watch fixed, and to the library for a gardening book. So I visualized myself driving down the parkway past the swimming pool to the mall where the jeweler and the hardware store are located. I then pictured myself buying a new rake and handing my watch to the jeweler. Next I imagined myself leaving the mall and driving through the busy downtown area to the library. Finally I visualized myself checking out a colorful book on gardening. It took much less time to visualize all this than I thought, under a minute. I was pleasantly surprised that this technique was so easy and useful.

(You may think, "That's too much work. I'll just make a list of my errands on a piece of paper or make a note in my phone." But we encourage you to give visualization a try, because it can be so useful. For example, you may think of a new errand while you are driving and not able to add an errand to your written or electronic list when it occurs to you.)

✳ EXERCISE: VISUALIZATION

Create a visual image to help you remember the following:

1. Mrs. Hammerman's name

_____

_____

_____

2. The car model called the Accord

_____

_____

_____

3. Parkinson's disease

_____

_____

_____

4. Lane 5B in a parking lot

_____

_____

_____

5. Buying a new windshield wiper blade while at the gas station

_____

_____

_____

See page 151 for possible answers.   ✱

Active Observation: Actively Observe and Think about What You Want to Remember.

It's often difficult to remember things that you haven't looked at carefully or with much interest. Active observation is the process of consciously paying attention to the details of what you see, hear, or read. By using active observation, you can find meaning and vibrancy in a photograph, a new face, a nature scene, a conversation, an occurrence on the street, or a piece of artwork. Active observation contrasts with passively letting life go on around you without much thought or interest. To actively observe a subject think about the meaning of the subject, how you feel about it, how it affects you, and whether you want to remember it. Ask yourself questions that will reinforce its meaning. A key to remembering anything is being interested in it.

This technique can be used to remember such things as

- The design of a quilt you saw in a store (you can also use your smartphone or digital camera to record the quilt design)
- The way to play a new game your friend is teaching you
- The faces of people you see in the hallway of your apartment complex
- The difference between a fir tree and a juniper

EXAMPLES

Steve: I parked in a parking garage at a shopping mall. There were several up and down ramps on each level and no letters or numbers designating the area where I parked. I realized that I could easily misplace my car. I carefully observed the route I took to the exit stairway and, when I got there, looked back to reinforce the image of the location of my car. When I returned several hours later, I had a strong visual memory of where my car was located and how to get there.

Jane: I went to our local museum and spent some time looking at a painting of two women by Monet. Instead of just glancing at the painting as I usually do, I looked at the details as well as the whole painting and asked myself some questions: Did I think it was beautiful? What time of year was it? Did the women look happy or sad? What were they wearing? Was there anything unusual about the painting? Would I like to have it hanging in my living room? When I left the museum, I knew that I would remember that painting. This trip to the museum would be more than just the usual blur of pictures.

✽ EXERCISE: ACTIVE OBSERVATION

Look at the picture below, consciously paying attention to the details. Ask yourself questions about the picture's meaning and its effect on you as you look at it.

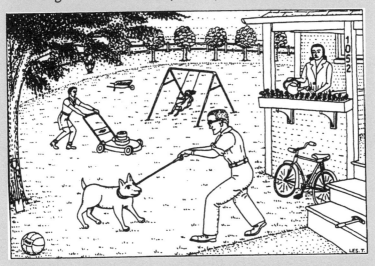

Now, cover the picture and see if you can answer these questions:

How many people are in the picture?
What is the boy doing?
What is the woman doing?
What is leaning against the house?
What is on the steps?
What is the number on the house?
What is the man doing?

If you are able to answer most of these questions, you have used excellent powers of observation.   ✽

Elaboration: Elaborate on the Details of the Information You Want to Remember.

A brief and unexamined thought is fragile and easily forgotten. But when we elaborate on the details of the thought, we encode the idea more deeply. We experience this depth of processing unintentionally when something interesting or controversial occurs, such as a bridge collapse. Without recognizing what we are doing, we comment on an unusual occurrence in our minds: we try to understand what happened; we relate it to what we know of the situation; we ask ourselves how we feel about it. This process of elaboration, which happens unconsciously in unusual circumstances, can be used intentionally as a strategy for encoding even everyday information that we want to remember.

Try this technique if you want to remember such things as

- The instructions for using your new espresso machine
- The platforms of the two mayoral candidates
- The courses that your son is taking in college
- The directions to the new recreation building
- The plot of a book you want to discuss with a friend

EXAMPLES

John: I recently got a new smartphone. I decided that I wanted to keep my calendar on the phone. My son showed me briefly how to do it. When I got back home and started to transfer my paper calendar to my phone, I realized that I had forgotten what he said. The next time I saw my son, I asked him to show me again. While we were still together, I talked myself through the steps, repeated his instructions a couple of times aloud, and practiced it. After elaborating on the details of this task, I found that when I returned home, I could do it on my own.

Jill: I took the trip of a lifetime to the Hawaiian Islands. I visited three of the islands—all of which are gorgeous and different from each other. I wanted to be able to talk about the islands without mixing them up. I had read in the newspaper that if you elaborate on the details of what you want to remember, you will encode the information more deeply. I thought about the different physical characteristics of the island, what I did on each island, and where I stayed. I made some associations between these details and the names of the islands. For several days I repeated these details, and now I find it easy to remember.

✳ EXERCISE: ELABORATION

Every state has a nickname. Here are the nicknames of three states:

Minnesota: The Gopher State
Missouri: The Show Me State
Montana: The Treasure State

See if you can use elaboration to encode these states and their nicknames so that you can remember them tomorrow. When you wake up tomorrow, ask yourself if you can remember this information. If not, try elaborating on it more fully. (You will probably automatically use visualization to remember these nicknames as well.)   ✳

Repetition

Have you ever needed to keep something in your working memory long enough so you can act on it? Have you ever wanted to reinforce some information so that it is more easily available to you?

Repetition is a useful strategy for remembering such things as:

- The thing you wanted to get in another room
- A song you hear and want to add to your playlist
- The title of a book you hear reviewed on the radio while driving
- The instructions for doing a task with sequential steps
- The names of people you will be seeing at a gathering
- The items you want to get from the store

EXAMPLES

Patty enjoys walking around her neighborhood. She knows most of the people in the homes she passes but often can't recall their names. She begins naming the families in the homes as she passes each house, and through repetition, she reinforces the information.

Rob spends a lot of time on his computer. He is learning to use Photoshop. As he works on resizing photos, he repeats the sequential steps until it becomes an automatic process.

Natasha is on the way to a New Year's Eve party. She knows the names of all her friends who will be there but wants to be sure she can greet them all by the correct name. On the way to the gathering, she repeats the names so they are fresh in her mind.

16

You Don't Have to Keep Everything in Your Head

Always carry a notebook. And I mean always . . .
unless it is committed to paper you can lose an idea
for ever.

—Will Self

Although there are times when we have to rely on our memory for remembering, most people also use external reminders to prompt them throughout their daily lives. For example, we may keep a record of appointments on a paper or smartphone calendar, make grocery lists, use an oven timer for baking cookies, and rely on a pillbox that has compartments marked with the days and times of day. You probably agree that there is no need to trust your memory in these situations. If you can use something in your environment to cue yourself, your mind is free to think of other things. The following three external techniques may be familiar to you, but this chapter may help you adapt them in new ways.

Written Reminders: Write Things Down.

Is it a crutch to rely on lists, calendars, appointment books, and notes to keep track of what we want to remember? Absolutely not. Writing things down is one of the most useful memory tools around. It's best to keep all reminders in one notebook which you always return to a permanent and prominent place, like the kitchen counter, your pocket or purse, or a bedside table. Paper notebook or smart device? Or both? It's up to you.

The following list will give you ideas for creatively using written reminders in everyday life.

- Keep a running list of things you need to do. As soon as you think of something, add it to the list.
- Use your notebook or calendar to remind yourself of calls you want to make in the future, such as phoning a friend after an operation.
- Keep a list of health questions you want to ask your health provider at your next appointment. Write down your provider's instructions before you the leave the office.
- Keep a record of when you've written a letter or made an important phone call.
- Keep a list of books you want to read or books you have read.
- Record the name and dosage of each of your medications. Include the date you began taking it. Update this list every time you have a medication change of any kind.
- Make lists of people whose names you want to remember, such as neighbors, members of a social group, or children of your friends.
- Record the dates of events you would like to recall, such as your niece's birthday, the day and year of your daughter's wedding, or the anniversary of the death of your friend's husband. Record these dates on your calendar at the start of every year. Use the repeat option on an electronic calendar to automatically add these dates every year.
- The requirements for passwords vary considerably, and some of them are very complicated. Keep a list of your

passwords for online banking, travel websites, work sites, email, credit cards, shopping sites, smart devices, and so on. Keep this information in a private, secure place.

❋ ASSIGNMENT
_____

Within the next three days, set up a notebook that you will use to record whatever you might want to remember. Keep a record for one week and see if you find it helpful.

For example:

Diary

Paid car insurance, 6/29
sent package to Jane, 7/1
7/4 met new neighbor—Jack

To Do List

Buy thread
Call plumber 769-1130
watch TV special
on S. Africa   9:00

❋

One more thing about writing things down: A friend of ours, whose memory is quite impaired, is able to keep track of the events of her life by jotting down daily occurrences as they happen. Her notebook reminds her of events and visitors, and she is able to tell others how her day has gone.

Auditory Reminders: Use Sound to Trigger Your Memory.

You can use alarm clocks, timers, smartphones, and computers to remind yourself of something that must be done at a specific time in the future. A telephone answering machine can also be used to provide an auditory cue. Here are some ways to use auditory reminders.

- If you make a phone call and don't get through to the person, set a timer to remind yourself to call again.
- If you are away from home and want to remember to do something when you return, leave yourself a message on your answering machine or send yourself a text message.
- If you worry that you might lose track of time and be late to pick up a child from school, use a timer as a reminder.
- Smartphones have repeat alarm settings that can remind you to take your medicine each day at a certain time.
- If you're busy writing e-mail messages or surfing the Web and want to be sure to leave for an appointment at a specific time, set the calendar on your computer to send you a reminder message.

Environmental Change: Change Something in Your Surroundings So It Jogs Your Memory.

One of the most effective and easiest ways to remind yourself of a specific task is to change something in your environment so you notice the change. The change then serves as a cue to jog your memory. You must make the change as soon as you think of the task, however! Here are examples of environmental cues that would jog your memory.

- Set the clothes to take to the cleaners in front of the door you will leave by.
- Put a note on the kitchen table so you'll see it when you eat breakfast and remember to send a card to your aunt.
- Attach a note to the steering wheel to remind yourself to vote or stop at the hardware store.
- Tie a string around the handles of your purse so you can't open it without being reminded to mail the letter that's inside.
- When you're in the basement, put a waste basket or a simple sign in front of the stairway to remind yourself to turn off the heater before you go upstairs.
- Change your watch or ring to the other hand; you will constantly feel it. As you drive to your friend's house, it will remind you to tell him about the change in plans for the weekend. If you say aloud, "Tell Mario about the change in plans," the technique will work even better.

EXAMPLE

Peggy says, "It's easy to remember to silence my cell phone during a meeting or movie, but it's hard for me to remember to turn the ringer back on." She wondered what she could change in her environment to remind herself. She asked her friends, who came up with several ideas: change your ring or watch to the other hand; make a small X on your wrist with a pen; set the timer on your cell phone to the time the event will be over; tie a string around your finger or a put rubber band on your wrist. If you usually keep your cell phone in the pocket close to your dominant hand, move it to the pocket on the other side when you turn the ringer off. People who silence their phones at night can put a sticky note on the phone for a morning reminder.

When using any external memory aids, it is crucial to avoid procrastination. As soon as you think of something you need to do in the future, choose one of these techniques and act on it. If you think, "I'll move the clothes for the dry cleaner to the front door when this TV show is over," there's a chance you may forget about the clothes in the ten minutes it takes for the show to end.

We use external reminders all the time; still, glitches can occur. Here's what happened to one of us the other day. Lynn put her library book on the passenger seat of the car to remind her to return it to the library. When she offered a friend a ride, she moved the book to the back seat. Without the cue, she never thought about the book again until she got an overdue notice.

✳ EXERCISE: ENVIRONMENTAL CHANGE

Think of ways to jog your memory for the following tasks by using environmental change.

1. You want to remember to take your laptop to the office tomorrow.

   _____

   _____

   _____

2. You are out grocery shopping and want to remember to call your dentist when you get home.

   _____

   _____

   _____

3. You are at your exercise class and a friend asks you to bring a certain book to next week's class.

_____

_____

_____

4. You want to remember to put out the garbage tomorrow.

_____

_____

_____

5. You are sitting in a meeting and you remember that you have to stop at the store on your way home.

_____

_____

_____

See page 151 for possible solutions.   ✳

17
Did I or Didn't I?

Most people, probably, are in doubt about certain matters ascribed to their past. They may have seen them, may have said them, done them, or they may only have dreamed or imagined they did so.

—William James

We do many daily tasks so automatically that we don't pay much attention to them. If you worry about whether you turned off the stove, shut down the computer, or locked the door, you can use the technique of self-instruction.

Self-Instruction: Give Yourself Verbal Instructions about What You Want to Remember.

We do some things so automatically that it is easy to forget whether we did them. If you often ask yourself, "Did I remember to do that?" this technique is for you. As you lock the door, use self-instruction. If you say out loud to yourself, "I am now locking the door," you won't have to get out of bed later, to check.

This technique is powerful because it focuses your attention, which makes it much more likely that you will remember that you did indeed do the task. Here are situations where using this technique can save needless worry.

Did I?

Turn off the stove/iron/coffeepot/heater/computer
Lock the door
Make the phone call
Charge the cell phone
Adjust the thermostat
Order the book at the library
Reserve the conference room at work
Take my medicine
Turn off the basement light or front porch light
Book a table at the restaurant
Close the garage door
Water the plants
Stop the mail/newspaper

EXAMPLE

Dhara: I travel a lot for work and often, after leaving on a trip, I would ask myself whether I had remembered to adjust the thermostat for an empty house. In a book on memory, I learned that I should say out loud, "There. I just turned the thermostat down (or up)." I gave it a try and now I always add something like, "Good. I won't wonder if I'm sending money up the chimney while I'm out of town."

✳ ASSIGNMENT

For the next week, use self-instruction whenever you perform a task that might cause you to ask later, "Did I do that?" At the end of the week, notice whether using this technique was helpful. ✳

18

Remembering More
Than One Thing

Memory, my dear Cecily, is the diary that we all carry
about with us.

—*Oscar Wilde*

Have you ever gone to the store to buy three items and only
remembered two of them? This chapter describes helpful techniques for when you have several items to remember.

The Story Method: Devise a One-Sentence Story That Will Connect Things You Want to Remember.

The story method is the process of making up a simple yet vi-
brant sentence connecting items that seem to have no connection. Many people resist this technique because it strikes them
as either silly or complicated. We believe that if you give it a
try you will find it amazingly effective. This technique can be
used to remember such things as

- Two phone calls that you need to make when you get home
- Three things you want to tell your daughter when you
  call her

- Three items you need to pick up at the hardware store
- Two books you want to get at the library

In the following two examples, you may also need to use environmental change in addition to the story method.

EXAMPLES

You wake up in the night and start thinking of what you need to do the next day. You want to remember that you need to call your dentist, return a rug to the department store, and buy filters for the furnace, but you don't want to get out of bed to write a list. You make up a story connecting these items by visualizing your dentist using a rug to keep himself warm because his furnace broke down.

Now you need to change your environment in some way to remind yourself in the morning that you have created this story. How about moving your book from the night stand to the foot of your bed? Or putting your extra pillow on the floor?

You have to go to the cleaners and post office before you go home. You might make up a story about putting your pants into the mailbox and the chaos that would follow. How will you remember that you need to stop at all? How about moving your watch or ring to the other hand? Or you could put a note on your car keys or a rubber band around your wrist.

✳ EXERCISE: THE STORY METHOD

Make up a one- or two-sentence story connecting the following items.

1. Getting a duplicate key made, picking up a birthday cake, and going to the bank

_____

_____

_____

2. Shopping for stationery, cologne, and a broom

_____

_____

_____

See page 152 for possible solutions.   ✳

Chunking: Chunk Individual Numbers into a Group.

It's difficult for most people to remember long numbers. When you are trying to remember a group of numbers, look for ways to combine them. This technique can be used to remember such things as

- Phone numbers
- Street addresses and zip codes
- Social Security and driver's license numbers

EXAMPLES

You want to remember a local telephone number, such as 313-663-4735. You probably already know the area codes in your community and can group the seven numbers into four chunks, 66-34-7-35, which are easier to remember.

A driver's license or Social Security number has standard groupings, such as 343-49-4296. This number may be easier to remember if you change the "chunks" into 3-43-49-42-96 or 34-34-94-29-6 or 343-494-296.

✳ EXERCISE: CHUNKING

Memorize your driver's license number or Social Security number by experimenting with chunking the individual numbers. Analyze the sequence to see which way of chunking makes the most sense.   ✳

First-Letter Cues: Group the First Letters of a Series of Items.

This technique involves using the first letters of a list of words to form either another word or a meaningful sentence whose words begin with the same letters as the words on the list. Although this technique is hard to describe, it's easy to use. The following examples will give you the idea.

EXAMPLES

If you want to remember the names of the five Great Lakes, you can take the first letter of each lake and create the word HOMES (Huron, Ontario, Michigan, Erie, Superior).

Suppose you want to remember the name of each of the presidents from Nixon to Obama (Nixon Ford Carter Reagan Bush Clinton Bush Obama). You can take the first letter of each name and form a sentence that has meaning to you. Examples are:

Nine furry cats ran by curious baby owls.

or

News from cereal reviewers: Be cool, buy oatmeal.

You are driving in your car and think of four items you want from the grocery store but don't want to stop to write them down. You need beef, apples, a lemon, and milk. The first letters of these four items can form the word "lamb," which will serve as a memory cue. If the items do not form a word, try making a sentence with matching first letters. For example, if your list is soup, chicken, soap, and lettuce, you could create the sentence "Soapy chickens like soup" (or "Soupy chickens like soap!").

✳ EXERCISE: FIRST-LETTER CUES

1. Create a word or sentence using the first letters of the names of these downtown streets to help you remember them in order. In this case, it's important to keep the letters in the same order as the streets.

Main
Adams
Lincoln
Rose
Brown

2. Try using this technique to remember the names of
   your friend's cats.

Radar
Alice
Chloe

See page 152 for possible solutions.   ✳

Create a Word: Expand Random Letters into a Familiar Word.

Sometimes you need to remember a group of letters that
make no inherent sense, such as license plates or corporate
names. In this case you can add more letters, often vowels, to
form a familiar word.

EXAMPLES

On a license plate, you might form the word "extra" out of
"xra" or "lefty" out of "lft."

If you have trouble remembering the name of the company
that manages your apartment building, PND, expand these
letters to form the word "panda."

✳ EXERCISE: CREATE A WORD

Expand the following letters into words:

1. PLM _____
2. RBT _____
3. GLW _____
4. STR _____
5. HLD _____

See page 152 for possible solutions.   ✳

Categorization: Group a List of Items by Category.

Categorization is the process of looking at a random list of items and seeing how to group them by category. It is easier to remember three categories that serve as cues for several of the items in the list than to remember each of the nine items separately.

EXAMPLES

These nine items could be grouped into three categories:

Popcorn	Soda	Green chilies
Tuna	Cookies	Milk
Chips	Juice	Cranberry sauce

Canned goods: green chilies, cranberry sauce, tuna
Snacks: popcorn, chips, cookies
Liquids: milk, juice, soda

Imagine that you are trying to come up with a list of friends and acquaintances for an anniversary party. You might consider categories of friends, such as neighbors, work colleagues, church members, or card-playing friends. This technique would help you recall a larger number of your friends and acquaintances than a random thought process would.

✳ EXERCISE: CATEGORIZATION

Categorize the following items:

Broom	Mop	Scotch tape
Envelopes	Dish soap	Glue
Sponge	Furniture polish	Bleach

_____ .

_____ .

_____ .

See page 152 for possible solutions.   ✳

19

Improving Your Ability to Recall

I remembered that, and, remembering that, I
remembered everything.

—Neil Gaiman

Everyone needs help from time to time recalling information—
even when we know that information very well. When you
know that the information you seek is in your long-term memory but you can't recall it when you need it, there are three
helpful techniques to turn to.

Cue Yourself: Search Your Memory Bank for Related Facts That May Serve as Cues.

When you can't think of something that you know is stored
in your long-term memory, you may find that merely thinking longer and harder does not bring it back to mind. You
might try this instead. When you want to retrieve specific information from long-term memory, try thinking of related
facts. These facts may serve as cues to trigger the information you want.

129

This technique can be used for recalling

- The name of a famous person
- The French word for "friend"
- The name of a TV show
- Where an out-of-town friend lives
- What you did last Saturday

EXAMPLES

Betsy was on her way to the library to get a DVD of her grand-children's favorite show, because they were coming for a visit. She thought she would recognize the title in the children's section. When she got there, she discovered that there were hundreds of titles in that section, arranged alphabetically. Rather than spend her time working her way from A to Z in this section, she thought, "I should be able to come up with this title." She began to search for cues that would trigger the name of the program. Betsy thought about the main character wearing a stethoscope and remembered that she was a doctor. She thought, "It is Doc Something . . . Of course! It's *Doc McStuffins.*"

Jamie: I met a woman at a party last week. When she introduced herself, I knew I had met her before. I remembered our interaction, but I couldn't remember where we had met. After I left the party, I searched for cues related to our initial meeting that would trigger the information about where we met. I thought about how long ago the initial meeting took place, what we had talked about, who else was involved in the conversation, and my feelings about the interaction. It suddenly occurred to me that we had met at a fundraiser given by a coworker.

✳ EXERCISE: CUE YOURSELF

See if you can recall the two candidates who ran for president of the United States in 2000. If you don't immediately know, search your memory for related facts that could serve as cues for this information.

See page 153 for the answer.   ✳

Alphabet Search: Go through the Alphabet to Jog Your Memory.

Alphabet search is the process of thinking through the sounds of the letters of the alphabet from A to Z to see if one will serve as a cue to jog your memory.

EXAMPLES

If you're trying to remember the name of someone you have just met, run through the sounds of the alphabet. Hearing the sound of the letter "m" may trigger the name Mike.

You want to describe the food you ate last night to a friend but can't remember the word "fettucini." You might go through the alphabet hoping that the beginning sound of one of the letters will cue your memory.

✳ EXERCISE: LETTER CUES

Below you will find a column listing categories. Each category is followed by a letter. See if you can find a word that fits the category and begins with the corresponding letter.

Fruit with a P (for example, plum)
Animal with a D
Metal with an I
Bird with a B
Country with an F
Boy's name with an H
Girl's name with an A
Vegetable with a P
Weapon with an S
Flower with a P

Here is the same column of categories followed by letters, but this time, find a word that fits the category and ends with the corresponding letter.

Fruit with an H (for example, peach)
Animal with a W
Metal with an R
Bird with an N
Country with a Y
Boy's name with a D
Girl's name with an N
Vegetable with a T
Weapon with a W
Flower with a T

(Exercise adapted with permission from Alan Baddeley, *Your Memory: A User's Guide*, New York, Macmillan, 1982.)

See page 153 for possible answers.   ✳

Review in Advance: Review in Advance What You May Be Called upon to Remember.

Everyone knows the feeling of forgetting familiar information, such as a friend's name or a well-known author. When you have to recall this type of information on demand, it sometimes takes a few seconds to bring it to mind—just long enough to cause a mental block. This experience is especially likely if you are asked to recall something or someone you haven't thought about for a while. When you know you will be called upon to remember certain names or information, reviewing ahead of time will optimize your chances of remembering.

This technique can be used to help you keep in mind

- The relationships of the family members you will be seeing at the reunion
- The history of your medical problems when you see your doctor
- The things you want to talk with your son about when you take him to lunch
- The names of people you will be seeing at the annual meeting of your condominium association

EXAMPLES

If you are afraid you will not remember people's names at a family reunion or other gathering, prepare ahead of time by going over a list of everyone who might attend. Writing down the names and saying them out loud is more effective than simply reading through a list. As you say the name, visualize the person and something special about him or her, like red hair or a great laugh.

If you are going to a meeting of your book club, record the title of the book, the author, the names of characters, and your feelings about the book, and review your notes before you go. You might also find it helpful to read a review of the book online the day before the meeting.

If you are going to lunch with a friend, review the names of your friend's children and what you know about them beforehand, so you can ask your friend about them easily.

✳ ASSIGNMENT

Think of the next group meeting you will attend (exercise class, monthly poetry class, ski club, your partner's work party), or try to think of the names of the people who live near you. List the names below and review them several times. If you have trouble listing all of them at one time, add to the list as the names come to you.

_____

_____

_____

_____

_____

_____

_____

After you have completed this exercise, consider whether the review helped you remember the names more easily. Did this technique work for you?   ✷

20

General Tips for Remembering

I remember my childhood names for grasses and secret flowers. I remember where a toad may live and what time the birds awaken in the summer—and what trees and seasons smelled like—how people looked and walked and smelled even.

—John Steinbeck

1. **Believe in yourself.** Don't let negative expectations defeat you. If you expect to fail, you won't even try. If you find yourself thinking, "I can't remember names," substitute "I may forget some names, but by using memory improvement techniques I can do better."

2. **Make conscious choices about what you want to remember.** No one can remember everything. So put effort and energy into the areas that are most important to you.

3. **Focus your attention on what you really want to remember.** Much of what is called "forgetting" is a lack of attention. Before you blame your memory, ask yourself if you were really paying attention.

4. **Cut out distractions.** You may find it difficult to pay attention to more than one thing at a time. Recognize the

137

limitations of working memory, and cut out distractions whenever possible.

5. **Give yourself plenty of time.** People of all ages forget more frequently when they are rushing. In general, if you have enough time to think about what you need to accomplish, you are less likely to forget something. You may also find that you need more time for learning new information and for recalling information from long-term memory. Give yourself a little additional time and see if it helps in encoding and retrieving information.

6. **Use all of your senses.** Use as many senses as possible when you want to remember something well. When you say something aloud, you hear the sound. When you write something down, you see the words and feel the pen or pencil moving on the paper. If you want to remember the size or shape of something, use your sense of touch. Smell and taste are very powerful in triggering memories from long ago.

7. **Be organized.** The old saying "A place for everything, and everything in its place" is good advice for memory improvement. Make a decision to improve your organizational skills in whatever ways are important to you. If you routinely put your bills, keys, glasses, and wallet in the same place, you will not waste time searching for them.

8. **Recognize and deal with the factors that may be negatively affecting your memory.** In this book, we have discussed factors that can affect the memory process for people of all ages. As you grow older, you may experience more of these negative influences. Think about which factors might be affecting your memory, and look for possible solutions or ways to compensate.

9. **Ask for clarification.** If you're not sure you fully understand what someone says, ask for further details. When you

misunderstand information, it is encoded incorrectly. Don't be reluctant to admit that you don't understand.

10. Relax. Tension interferes with the memory process; relaxing often lets the memory come to the surface. When you feel anxious about the possibility of forgetting, you may become preoccupied with the anxiety and unable to concentrate on recalling the needed information. The solution is to take a deep breath and relax; frequently the information will come to you.

11. Laugh. Laughter breaks the tension of forgetting and keeps a memory lapse in perspective. When you start to tell a friend about a book you are reading and can't remember the title or when you begin to introduce your niece and can't come up with her name, admit that the word or name just escaped your mind, and laugh. Everyone has had that experience and can empathize.

12. Enjoy past memories. Recognize the richness of your storehouse of memories. You can experience great pleasure from recalling the events and people that have made up the fabric of your life. Life review can put the past and present into perspective. Take pride in your ability to remember the past and make it come alive for yourself and others.

Appendix
Alzheimer's Disease and Related Dementias

About Alzheimer's Disease

Alzheimer's (AHLZ-high-merz) disease is a progressive brain disorder that gradually destroys a person's memory and ability to learn, reason, make judgments, communicate, and carry out daily activities. As Alzheimer's progresses, individuals may also experience changes in personality and behavior, such as anxiety, suspiciousness, or agitation, as well as delusions or hallucinations.

Causes of Alzheimer's Disease

In the vast majority of cases, the cause of Alzheimer's disease remains unknown. Most experts agree that Alzheimer's, like other common and chronic conditions, likely develops as a result of multiple genetic and nongenetic factors rather than a single cause. Age is the greatest risk factor for Alzheimer's. Most Americans with Alzheimer's disease are age sixty-five or older.

A small percentage (about one percent) of Alzheimer's cases is caused by rare, genetic variation. In these inherited forms of Alzheimer's, the disease tends to strike younger individuals.

141

When Alzheimer's is first recognized in a person under age sixty-five, this is referred to as "younger-onset Alzheimer's."

Age, family history, and genetics are all risk factors we can't change. One promising line of research suggests that strategies for overall healthy aging may help keep the brain healthy and may even offer some protection against Alzheimer's. These measures include eating a healthy diet, staying socially active, avoiding tobacco and excess alcohol, and exercising both body and mind. What is good for your heart is also good for your brain, so monitoring heart disease, diabetes, stroke, high blood pressure, and high cholesterol is important.

What is the difference between Alzheimer's disease and normal age-related memory difficulties?

Activity	A person with memory problems	A person with typical age-associated memory changes
Forgets	Whole experiences	Parts of an experience
Remembers later	Rarely	Often
Can follow written or spoken directions	Gradually unable	Usually able
Can use notes	Gradually unable	Usually able
Can care for self	Gradually unable	Usually able

Source: *Caring for People with Alzheimer's Disease: A Manual for Facility Staff,* by Lisa P. Gwyther (Washington, DC: American Health Care Association and Alzheimer's Association, 2001).
Note: Determination of whether memory loss is associated with Alzheimer's disease can only be made by health care professionals.

How Does Alzheimer's Disease Affect the Brain?

Scientists believe that whatever triggers Alzheimer's disease begins to damage the brain years before symptoms appear.

When symptoms emerge, nerve cells that process, store, and retrieve information have already begun to degenerate and die. Scientists regard two abnormal microscopic structures called "plaques" and "tangles" as the hallmarks of Alzheimer's disease. Amyloid plaques (AM-uh-loyd plaks) are clumps of protein fragments that accumulate outside of the brain's nerve cells. Tangles are twisted strands of another protein that form inside brain cells. Scientists have not yet determined the exact role that plaques and tangles may play.

Diagnosing Alzheimer's Disease

Although Alzheimer's symptoms can vary widely, the first problem that many people notice is forgetfulness severe enough to affect performance at home, at work, or in favorite activities. Sometimes the decline in memory may be more obvious to a family member or close friend than to the affected individual. Other common symptoms include confusion, getting lost in familiar places, and difficulty with language. The Alzheimer's Association encourages everyone who notices these symptoms in themselves or someone close to them to consult a physician.

A skilled physician can diagnose Alzheimer's disease with 90 percent accuracy. Because there is no single test for Alzheimer's, diagnosis usually involves a thorough medical history and physical examination as well as tests to assess memory and the overall function of the mind and nervous system. The physician may ask a family member or close friend about any noticeable change in the individual's memory or thinking skills.

One important goal of the diagnostic workup is to determine whether symptoms may be due to a treatable condition. Depression, medication side effects, certain thyroid conditions, excess use of alcohol, and nutritional imbalances are all potentially treatable disorders that may sometimes impair memory or other mental functions. Even if the diagnosis is Alzheimer's, timely identification enables individuals to take an active role in treatment decisions and planning for the future.

Alzheimer's is the leading cause of dementia, a group of conditions that all gradually destroy brain cells and lead to progressive decline in mental function. Most diagnostic uncertainty arises from occasional difficulty distinguishing Alzheimer's disease from one of these related disorders.

Other Causes of Dementia

Vascular dementia results from damage caused by multiple strokes within the brain. Symptoms can be similar and can even coincide with Alzheimer's disease and may include disorientation, confusion, and behavioral changes.

Normal pressure hydrocephalus (NPH) is a rare disease caused by an obstruction in the flow of spinal fluid leading to a buildup of fluid in the brain. Symptoms include difficulty in walking, memory loss, and incontinence. NPH may be related to a history of meningitis, encephalitis, or brain injury and is occasionally correctable with surgery.

Parkinson's disease affects the control of muscle activity, resulting in tremors, stiffness, and speech difficulties. In late stages, dementia can occur. Parkinson's drugs can improve steadiness and control but have no effect on mental deterioration.

Dementia with Lewy bodies is a disorder that, although progressive, is often initially characterized by wide variations in attention and alertness. Affected individuals often experience visual hallucinations as well as muscle rigidity and tremors similar to those associated with Parkinson's disease.

Huntington's disease is a fatal, progressive, hereditary disorder characterized by irregular movements of the limbs and facial muscles, a decline in thinking ability, and personality changes.

Frontotemporal dementia, also known as Pick's disease, is a rare brain disease that closely resembles Alzheimer's, with personality changes and disorientation that may precede memory loss.

Creutzfeldt-Jakob disease (CJD) is a rare ultimately fatal disorder of infectious or genetic origin that typically causes memory failure and behavioral changes. A recently identified form called "variant Creutzfeldt-Jakob disease (vCJD)" is the human disorder thought to be caused by eating meat from cattle affected by "mad cow disease" (bovine spongiform encephalopathy). Variant CJD tends to appear in much younger individuals than those affected by sporadic or inherited Creutzfeldt-Jakob.

Treating Alzheimer's Disease

Currently, there is no cure for Alzheimer's and no way to stop the underlying death of brain cells. But drugs and nondrug treatments may help with both cognitive and behavioral symptoms. Two types of drugs are currently approved by the U.S. Food and Drug Administration (FDA) to treat cognitive symptoms of Alzheimer's disease.

One important part of treatment is supportive care that helps individuals and their families come to terms with the diagnosis, obtain information and advice about treatment options, and maximize quality of life through the course of the illness.

As the pace of research accelerates, scientists funded by the Alzheimer's Association, the pharmaceutical industry, universities, and our federal government have gained detailed understanding of the basic disease process at work in the Alzheimer brain. Experts believe that several of these processes may offer promising targets for a new generation of treatments to prevent, slow, or even reverse damage to nerve cells.

About the Alzheimer's Association

For more than thirty years, the Alzheimer's Association has provided reliable information, created supportive programs and services for families, increased resources for dementia research, and influenced changes in public policy. They are the world leader in Alzheimer research and support. Their goal is to create a powerful constituency of passionate Americans that places the prevention and cure of Alzheimer's disease at the top of its agenda. To learn more, please contact them at:

Contact Center: 800-272-3900
Website: www.alz.org
e-mail: info@alz.org

What Additional Resources Are Available?

The Alzheimer's Association is the trusted resource for reliable information, education, referral and support to the millions of people affected by the disease, their families and caregivers, and health care professionals.

- Their 24/7 Helpline, 800-272-3900, provides information, referrals and care consultations in more than 170 languages and dialects.
- Their website, alz.org, provides comprehensive information about Alzheimer's disease and how the association can help those affected.

- Their online Safety Center, alz.org/safety, features information, tips, and resources to assist you with safety inside and outside of the home, wandering and getting lost, and driving and dementia.
- Their support groups, conducted at hundreds of locations nationwide, provide people with Alzheimer's and their families a confidential open forum to share concerns and receive support.
- ALZConnected (alzconnected.org), powered by the Alzheimer's Association, is a social networking community that connects people living with Alzheimer's, their caregivers, and others affected by the disease.
- Alzheimer's Association Alzheimer's Navigator (alzheim ersnavigator.org) is an online assessment program that creates customized action plans while connecting the individual to local community programs, services, and resources.
- Education workshops led by trained professionals on topics such as caregiving, brain health, Alzheimer's basics, and living with dementia, as well as a number of free e-learning courses available at elearning.alz.org.
- The Alzheimer's Association Green-Field Library is the nation's largest resource center devoted to Alzheimer's disease and dementia.

Material on the Alzheimer's Association courtesy of the Alzheimer's Association, Michigan Great Lakes Chapter and is used with permission. Copyright © 2014.

Answers to the Exercises

Recall (page 20) and Recognition (page 28)

1. Springfield
2. Judy Garland
3. Gerald Ford
4. Rudolph Giuliani

Understanding the Memory Process (pages 29–30)

When you go to the library and see a lot of colorful books on the "new books" shelf, the component of memory you are using is **sensory input.** You read through the titles and think about whether they interest you. These conscious thoughts occur in the component of memory called **working memory.** Then you find a book by a favorite author, John Grisham. You take down the book, notice how long it is, read the back cover, think it sounds familiar, and decided that you have read this book before. This process is called **encoding.** The information about the book leaves your conscious thought and goes into the component of memory called **long-term memory,** where it may be available for **retrieval** at another time. When you get home, you notice another of Grisham's books on your nightstand. This favorite book serves as a **cue** to remind you of the book in the library. The connection between the library book and your book at home is called **association.**

How Memory Works (page 31)

1. F	4. T	7. F
2. F	5. T	
3. T	6. T	

Learning New Information (pages 44–45)

1. People who are depressed or anxious.
2. One example of a distorted thought is "I am worthless."
3. A depressed person is less likely to be active.
4. One problem-solving strategy is to break problems into small steps.

How Memory Changes (pages 49–50)

1. T	3. T	5. T
2. F	4. T	6. T

Factors That Affect Memory (page 89)

1. T	5. T	9. F
2. F	6. T	10. T
3. T	7. F	
4. F	8. T	

Association (pages 99–100)

1. Since you are going to the doctor, associate "west" with "wellness"—both words begin with W.
2. Associate 2008 with the fact that you were born in 1948. Or if you don't have a convenient birthdate, you could say, "*Eight* was the *End* of my working life."
3. Associate "Campbell" with Campbell's soup and "Rose" with the red of the label on the soup can. It may help to visualize her face on a Campbell's soup can.
4. Associate the name "Turner" with turning your health around. Say to yourself several times, "Turner turned my health around."

Visualization (pages 102–103)

1. Visualize a giant *hammer* hitting a *man*.
2. Imagine your car being towed with *a cord*.
3. Visualize a woman sitting in the *park* with the *sun* beating down on her shoulders.
4. Visualize *five balloons* tied to your car antenna.
5. Visualize yourself paying for a tank of gas and asking the attendant for a replacement windshield wiper.

Environmental Change (pages 114–115)

1. Put the laptop in front of the door as soon as you think about returning it.
2. Write yourself a note in big letters on the grocery bag so that when you unpack the groceries you'll see it.
3. Put a note in your purse or gym bag. When you unpack the bag or open the purse, you will be reminded of the book. As soon as you think of it, put the book with your exercise clothes or equipment. (You might also put the responsibility

back on the person who wants the favor, and ask her to text your cell phone or call your home phone and leave a message.)
4. Put a big sign on the bathroom mirror or on the kitchen counter.
5. Change your watch or ring to the other hand.

The Story Method (page 123)

1. Envision a birthday cake shaped like a safe. You use a key to open it and find a huge pile of money.
2. See yourself breaking the bottle of cologne and sweeping up the pieces into a box of stationery.

First-Letter Cues (pages 125–126)

1. Mother Always Liked Rose Best.
2. CAR or ARC

Create a Word (page 127)

1. Plum
2. Robot
3. Glow
4. String
5. Hold

Categorization (page 128)

Desk items	Cleaning tools	Cleaning products
Envelopes	Sponge	Dish soap
Scotch tape	Broom	Furniture polish
Glue	Mop	Bleach

Cue Yourself (page 131)

George W. Bush and Al Gore

Letter Cues (pages 132–133)

Beginning Letter

Fruit with a P: peach
Animal with a D: donkey
Metal with an I: iron
Bird with a B: bobolink
Country with an F: Finland
Boy's name with an H: Hank
Girl's name with an A: Anna
Vegetable with a P: parsnip
Weapon with an S: sword
Flower with a P: peony

Ending Letter

Fruit with an H: peach
Animal with a W: cow
Metal with an R: copper
Bird with an N: wren
Country with a Y: Hungary
Boy's name with a D: Rod
Girl's name with an N: Marion
Vegetable with a T: beet
Weapon with a W: bow and arrow
Flower with a T: violet

(Exercise adapted with permission from Alan Baddeley, *Your Memory: A User's Guide*, New York, Macmillan, 1982.)